While You Were Out

While You Were Out

AN INTIMATE FAMILY PORTRAIT OF
MENTAL ILLNESS IN AN ERA OF SILENCE

Meg Kissinger

CELADON
BOOKS

NEW YORK

For Danny, because he wanted us to understand

To live in this world

you must be able
to do three things:
to love what is mortal;
to hold it

against your bones knowing
your own life depends on it;
and, when the time comes to let it go,
to let it go

—MARY OLIVER, "IN BLACKWATER WOODS"

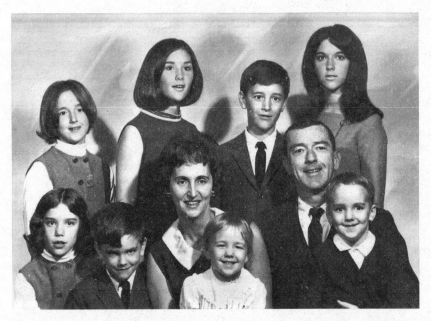

The Kissingers. Front row, from left: Patty, Billy, Molly on our mother's lap, and Danny on Holmer's lap. Back row: Meg, Nancy, Jake, and Mary Kay.

Contents

Author's Note

If any of my brothers or sisters pulled a stunt like this, I'd probably file a restraining order against them. There's a lot of tough stuff in this book that I can't imagine they are excited to see in print. Yet each has been helpful and encouraging as I spent years researching and writing it. They all agreed to be interviewed multiple times, often about the most traumatic and humiliating events of our lives. They've read what I've written and declared that it is accurate to the best of their knowledge.

I'm amazed by their magnanimity, but not surprised. In addition to freckles and crooked pinkie fingers, we share two signature traits: humor as a subversive form of coping and the willingness to lay ourselves bare to help others.

A note about accuracy: I'm an investigative reporter and journalism professor, trained to bulletproof my stories by verifying every fact with as much documentation and supporting evidence as possible. There was no way to do that here. Details come from letters, diaries, emails, police reports, coroners' reports, legal files, court transcripts, bankruptcy filings, army documents, census data, newspaper articles, and hundreds of pages of my family's medical records. I interviewed as many people as I could find with firsthand knowledge of the events I describe—doctors, social workers, family friends, neighbors, relatives, and lawyers. I even tracked down our old nanny from 1961 to 1963. She was a college student then and now lives in a retirement community in Florida.

Still, even the sharpest memories can be fuzzy. We were a family of eight children, born over a span of twelve years, to parents with serious illnesses who gobbled tranquilizers and drank themselves silly many nights. As you might imagine, there was a great deal of chaos in our house. I'm the fourth oldest, a pretty good perch from which to observe, but still prone to blind spots.

There's also the matter of trauma, which can mess with memory by erasing big chunks of time and freezing other parts disproportionately. So I can't swear that things happened in precisely the sequence that I describe with the same confidence that I bring to my journalism. I am careful to make note of those moments when they pop up throughout the book.

Any quotes included here are taken word for word from documents or taped interviews. Those drawn from memory or family stories—the ones I cannot swear were spoken verbatim—are included in italics without quotation marks.

Finally, my brother Billy wanted me to mention that he won the seventh-grade boys' basketball free throw contest *and* one-on-one tournament at St. Francis Xavier School in Wilmette, Illinois, in 1973. Other than that, no demands were made.

PART I

Loving What Is Mortal

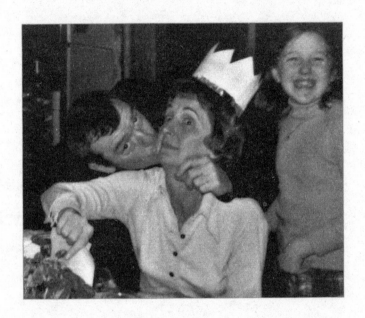

I
The Tiger Pit

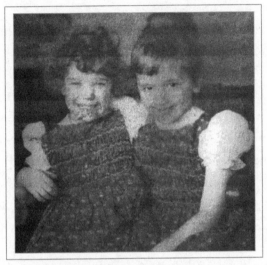

*Tiger Pit pals: Patty and me, dressed alike, as always,
for a party after Danny's baptism in
New Canaan, Connecticut, in 1963.*

When we were little, my sister Patty and I liked to pretend that ferocious tigers lurked in the space between our twin beds, just waiting to rip us to shreds. They stalked us at night with their razor-sharp fangs, growling and snorting and licking their chops. Dip a toe or a finger down too low and . . . *SNAP!* . . . they'd chomp it off clean to the bone. We'd bounce from one bed to the next, shrieking as we flew through the air.

Pipe down, you two, or I'll come in there and beat you to a bloody pulp! my mother would yell from her bedroom down the hall.

The invisible tigers scared us. Our mother did not.

Watch this, I'd whisper to Patty as I leaned over the side of my bed and slowly wiggled my fingers down into the pit. She'd poke her curly little head over the side of her bed and stare into the big black hole, nervously wheezing as she waited for one of the tigers to take the bait. I'd squeeze my eyes shut, imagining the hungry beasts skulking toward us, the smell of their musky fur filling my nostrils, and feel the thumping of my heart in the middle of my throat.

I said, "Pipe down!" my mother would call out, weaker this time.

We knew that she didn't have the energy to beat us, much less into any bloody pulp.

My mother, Jean Kissinger, an erstwhile debutante with a genius IQ, now spent her days rubbing ointment on babies' blistered bottoms, wiping snot off our faces, plastering our cowlicks with her spit, and dripping warm medicine into our oozing, infected ear canals. She stuffed our lunch bags with peanut-butter-and-potato-chip sandwiches as she helped us conjugate Latin verbs, folded laundry while she quizzed us on our multiplication tables, and typed our term papers between bouncing a baby on her lap and ironing our uniform blouses. Her own mother was dead and she had no sisters, so it fell to my mother to raise her eight children more or less by herself while my father was out of town most of the week on business.

My father, Bill Kissinger (we called him Holmer), sold advertising space to companies that manufactured tranquilizers and other so-called ethical pharmaceuticals to harried mothers of the baby boom. Business was brisk, especially in our North Shore Chicago neighborhood, where women, a great number of them Irish Catholics like my mother, were expected to fill the pews with as many children as they could bear, whether they had the stamina or not.

"Something is definitely wrong when the best that the average American couple can do over a fertile period of twenty-five years is to give only two or three children to the Kingdom of God," Monsignor John Knott of the National Catholic Welfare Conference said in his directive to the faithful.

The *Catholic Marriage Manual* that my mother and her friends read religiously cautioned, "When parents consciously choose the small family as their way of life, they are expressing their ambition for material luxury as opposed to the spiritual pleasures which child rearing can give. It is no coincidence that the 'spoiled little brat'—the selfish monster of popular fiction and newspaper comic strips—is usually an only child."

My mother might not have taken too kindly to these single men telling her how many children she should have and how to raise them, but she didn't do anything to contradict them. She and Holmer gamely produced five girls and three boys from 1952 to 1964, each one feistier than the last, scrapping and chasing and pawing like a pack of puppies. Our favorite game is one we made up called Teddy Bear. It starts with one kid jumping on top of another on the playroom floor. Then, one by one, the rest of us stack our bodies like human Jenga pieces, until someone farts or begins to turn blue. Meet the team:

1952, Mary Kay: The oldest. The arty one, glamorous and flamboyant, with thick dark brown hair that she would roll around orange juice cans each night to shape it just so. She spent hours transforming the room over our garage into a magic fairyland by gluing sparkles on the walls and dangling clumps of cotton from hangers to look like clouds.

Mary Kay was famous for her avant-garde fashions, often homemade. For her senior prom, she created earrings out of flashcubes and a white tunic with fringed sleeves like the brise-soleil from a Calatrava sculpture. Her "Jesus sandals" strapped around her legs up to her knees.

The first time she was grounded for staying out too late, Mary Kay decorated the back of her bedroom door with hundreds of pictures of eyes that she cut out of her *Seventeen* magazines, a *Great Gatsby* homage that I found to be as creepy as it was mesmerizing. She refused to go on our annual ski trips because she said her vacation was getting a week away from all of us. *I'm never getting married or having kids,* she'd say loudly and often enough to be sure that our mother heard her.

Hoping some of Mary Kay's swank would transfer to me by osmosis, I sometimes slept in the spare twin bed in her bedroom. After turning out the lights, she'd reach for the pack of Kool cigarettes that she'd hidden in a big green glass ashtray under her bed. As I watched the red glow from her cigarette dance through the darkness, I felt deliciously naughty to be in on an act of such insubordination.

1953, Nancy: The scamp. She was glamorous, too, but in a more conventional way that belied her truer nature. Nancy wore monogrammed blouses with pleated skirts and penny loafers with actual pennies tucked into the flaps. Both Mary Kay and Nancy modeled in high school and took the business of being beautiful very seriously. Every morning before school, those two would tie up the girls' bathroom, preening in front of the mirror, teasing their hair, gluing on false eyelashes, slathering on foundation and lip gloss. I could never figure out who they were trying to impress at their all-girls Catholic high school.

All right already! I'd whine as I danced around, waiting for them to finish the hell up so I could get to the toilet. Nancy played the piano and guitar and fancied herself the next Janis Joplin, wailing out soulful ballads of love gone wrong from the Kin-tucky coal mines to the California sun. It was hard to take her seriously. She sang off-key and, in her plaid wool shorts, Peter Pan collar, and gold circle pin, she looked nothing like the hipster, heroin-shooting blues singer. The nuns told my parents that Nancy was probably a genius, but to watch out: *She's sneaky.* Truer words were never spoken. Nancy and her friend Ellen won the school's eighth-grade science fair for their project on extrasensory perception, which meant they got to compete in the state contest in Springfield. The night before, Holmer caught Nancy changing the letters on the poster board from "ESP: Fact or Fiction?" to "Fuck on Fart."

This was the same year Nancy talked me into letting her pour a bottle of Clairol Summer Blonde dye on my hair. She was flirting with the notion of lightening her locks and figured I'd be the perfect guinea pig. After the chemicals turned my hair the color of an orangutan, Nancy aborted the mission. I was in fourth grade, and when my dark hair started growing back in, she loudly nicknamed me "Roots," a humiliating moniker that quickly spread around our grade school playground. At night, I used to sneak into her room and steal her sweaters. If she caught me, she'd scratch my arm or pull my orange hair.

1954, Jake: The observer/inventor. Fixated on efficiency, he combined salt and pepper into one shaker and would sometimes eat breakfast late at night in case he didn't have time to do so the next morning. Jake left notes he scribbled to my mother in the refrigerator to remind her, "Sliced cheese costs the same, tastes just as good, and is easier to use when making sandwiches." He filled plastic bags with ice and wore them around his neck on sultry summer days as he pedaled his bike toward Lake Michigan invoking his motto: *Under 75 degrees or underwater!*

Jake brought a backpack full of maps, almanacs, and little notebooks with him wherever we went and made pronouncements about modern culture that were impossible to prove. He'd say things like, *No one eats in their cars anymore* or *Catholics don't buy full-length mirrors.* He sounded authoritative enough, but if you asked for his sources, you'd find that they were anecdotal or based on very small sample sizes.

When Jake was in seventh grade, kids beat him up on the St. Francis playground so viciously that my parents transferred him to the public school. Not only had I done nothing to stop the harassment, I pretended not to notice. Once, I even laughed nervously. Like Peter in the garden at Gethsemane, I knew instantly that I had just betrayed the one person in my life who most consistently modeled love and compassion, and I was bitterly disappointed in myself for being so weak.

1957, Me: The bedrooms were full by the time I arrived. So, for the first several months, I slept in a bassinet by the front door like a human burglar alarm. From the few baby pictures taken of me, I can see why there weren't more. The left side of my face was swollen where the forceps had grabbed me, making it look like I was winking, the creepy way a prizefighter does after getting clobbered in the tenth round. My feet turned in toward each other, so I had to wear plaster casts on both legs and baby shoes affixed to a metal bar to keep them straight.

My mother worried about why I didn't walk or talk or reach for things as early as her other kids. The pediatrician examined me thoroughly and considered all the evidence. *You're right, Jean,* he told her. *This one is slow. But she'll probably be okay socially.*

1959, Patty: My wingman, a Goody Two-shoes who worked so hard to please me and everyone else that my friend Mary Claire nicknamed her Yygor (pronounced EE-gor), an eccentric spelling of Dr. Frankenstein's assistant. She baked pretzels for Holmer in her Easy-Bake oven and made a papier-mâché likeness of him one Father's Day, using one of his many empty beer bottles as the body.

With my stick-straight hair, I admit to being jealous when old ladies in the grocery store would coo at Patty's adorable ringlets. So I told her that she was adopted and her real parents were Malcolm X and a lady I made up named Kitty O'Shea. Patty had asthma, and on Christmas morning of 1961, when I was four years old and she was two, I sat on her chest— why, I do not recall—and she had to be rushed to the hospital while I hid under her bed, convinced that I'd murdered her.

Still, Patty was so cheerful and trustworthy that she was named editor of her first-grade newspaper, *The Happy Times.* She started keeping a diary, but maintained a strict policy of not reporting anything that might embarrass anyone or hurt their feelings. Before long, she ran out of news. By the following May, Patty abandoned journalism altogether and settled on a career in nursing.

1961, Billy: The golden boy—smart, funny, handsome, athletic, and a rascal of the first degree. His raspy voice was so appealing that Holmer once paid him a dollar just to hear him sing the ABCs. Billy and I would spend hours watching Chicago Cubs baseball games on our playroom TV, imitating pitchers' deliveries and batters' stances. When the score was close, we'd stand on one leg for good luck.

When he was in second grade, Billy tried to sneak a pack of my mother's cigarettes to school by zipping them into the front pocket of his windbreaker. He had a crush on his teacher that year and wore English Leather aftershave to woo her. That was the same year that his band of little hooligans lit the neighbor's woods on fire. Everyone assumed Billy would grow up to be a wild man like Holmer, his namesake.

1963, Danny: The youngest boy was born on Billy's second birthday, so the comparisons between the two were even more tempting. With his big, deep-set brown eyes, strawberry-blond hair, and rosy cheeks, Danny looked like a Gerber baby. He'd crawl around the playroom in his yellow Dr. Denton pajamas and curl up next to the radiator like a cat. Danny had such a sweet disposition that the manager of our local grocery store called him "the Good, Good Baby." We called him "Duper" or "the Dupe," for short. While Billy was running around the block naked with the little girl next door, the Dupe quietly strung rope around the necks of plastic army men he called "my guys" and dangled them from his third-floor bedroom window.

Danny aimed to please. He knew that my mother loved BLT sandwiches, so he taught himself how to make them for her. His mouth curled up on one side, making it look like he was always smiling. But I always worried about that little guy. You had to keep your eye on him or he'd find himself in more trouble than he could handle.

One summer day, when Danny was about three, he toddled out the back door while no one was looking. Patty and I canvassed the neighborhood on our bikes and found him eating grass behind the fence of an old lady's yard a few blocks away. *Let him go!* we screamed. But she shooed us away with her broom. We were convinced that she was a witch trying to fatten him up for the cauldron.

1964, Molly: The baby of the family didn't come home from the hospital right away because my mother refused to leave the maternity ward. She said she was too tired from having had all these kids and she needed to stay there for a while longer to get some rest. They arrived home just in time for my seventh birthday, so I assumed that Molly was a gift just for me. I used to take her out of her crib and bring her into my bed to sleep with me at night until she was old enough to roll over and fall out. *Stay little,* I would whisper into her ear as she slept. I didn't want her growing up and leaving me. My friends and I would come home from school and run into the nursery to wake her from her naps by chanting the silly nickname we gave her: *Roeger Boohead Boohead Hogmeier, sat in the crib all fat and bald!!!* Molly would stare at us through the slats of her crib and shout, *Gee-bo-shut!* which we eventually deciphered as *Get out of here* and *Shut up.*

Without any sisters near her in age, Molly lacked fashion sense. She wore the same polyester pants—navy blue with little moons—for several days in a row, even after they were too tight for her. More than once, Holmer accused Molly of peeing in our backyard swimming pool, a claim she never denied convincingly. But you could tell that he was proud of how she could drain a free throw, spike a volleyball, and swing a golf club. *She even farts like a man,* Holmer twinkled on the day Molly got her first hole in one.

MY PARENTS LIKELY WOULD have had more children, but even the parish priest agreed that enough was enough. By 1964, with her nerves frayed and her uterus all but shot, my mother went on the Pill. Her doctor, a Catholic and the father of ten, wrote the prescription. *Your body can't handle any more, Jean,* he told her, to say nothing of her mind.

My mother was taking quite a risk. Official Catholic doctrine held that all birth control—except for the famously ineffective rhythm method—goes against the natural order of God. Any woman who took the Pill would be committing a mortal sin. If she were caught, my mother would not just be denied Holy Communion for life, she would burn in hell for eternity. But a glimmer of hope for her salvation flickered in the distance. Theologians meeting at the Vatican were recommending that the pope allow oral contraception. The Pill doesn't destroy human life, they argued. It merely prevents it from forming by stopping ovulation. A decision could come any day.

As my mother awaited the verdict, she nervously swallowed her pill each morning. She was down in the basement doing one of her many daily loads of laundry when the news broke over the radio: Oral contraceptives are "intrinsically wrong," Pope Paul VI declared. They cannot be used as a means of regulating the number of children in a family. Any woman wishing to remain a Catholic in good standing may not take the Pill. Period. End of discussion.

Well, shit, my mother said.

She trudged upstairs to find a church bulletin, relieved to see that Father Welsh, the young associate, was assigned to hear confessions that week. Finally, a lucky break. Off she went to see him bright and early the following Saturday.

Father, it's me, Jean Kissinger, my mother whispered as she knelt in the darkened box. Hadn't she done enough to propagate the faith? The newly minted priest fumbled for a bit. *But, Jean,* he said. *Children are gifts from God, the fruits of a loving relationship.* Her heart sank. This new priest might not be such a pushover after all.

My mother was desperate. What began as mild postpartum depression after Jake was born grew more intense with each new baby and was now nearly paralyzing her. She was terrified of what might happen if she had to keep having children. By then, she was forty-two years old, the same age that her mother had been when she became pregnant with her youngest child, Johnny, who was born with Down syndrome.

Please, Father, my mother pleaded, *I can't have any more children.* She told him about her dark thoughts and how she wasn't always able to shake herself out of that funk. After a good, long while, the young priest conceded the point.

Okay, Jean, he said, *fair enough.* And he granted her the dispensation.

A week later, our home phone rang, and I answered. The normally chatty Father Welsh sounded peeved. He told my mother that the line of women waiting for his confessional that Saturday snaked all the way to the back of the church. Apparently, my mother couldn't keep her trap shut about the deal she'd finagled. Now all her friends were looking to get in on the action.

Jean, Father Welsh scolded, *what goes on in confession is private BOTH ways.*

EVEN THROUGH THE FOG of her depression and anxiety, my mother did her best to make our house a happy one. She'd start out strong each morning, padding around the kitchen in her fuzzy blue slippers, a Kent cigarette dangling from her lower lip, singing to Tippy, our fat beagle, and the canary we named Flip the Bird. She scribbled her lists of things to do that day on the back of a bank deposit slip. (First item: "Make List.") She wore a creamy pink Barbizon bathrobe with a Susan B. Anthony button pinned to her lapel that declared, "All Men Are Beasts."

Late mornings, once she'd taken her bath, she might head to St. Francis Xavier School for her turn at playground duty, breaking up fights, cleaning skinned knees, and making sure kids' coats were buttoned up against the stiff winds that blew off the shores of nearby Lake Michigan. After school, she would lug us around Chicago's North Shore in her wood-paneled station wagon while she ran errands or tended to one of her many corporal works of mercy. She delivered breast milk for the La Leche League and care packages of clothing, toys, and food that she'd assemble for the Cordi-Marian Society, the church's mission. When one of her friends had a baby or a parent who died, she'd make them her signature lemon bars. We'd wait in the car with the engine running while my mother scurried to the door to deliver any treats that were left after we'd raided the basement refrigerator the night before, ignoring the skulls and crossbones that she scrawled on her warning labels: DO NOT EAT!!!! 💀 💀 💀

After that, she would haul us to our basketball games or play practices or scout meetings where my mother often presided as leader. *Good enough*, she'd say, handing us our fitness badges as we turned lopsided somersaults and cartwheels. Then she'd schlep us over to the Hi-Lo Grocery store on Green Bay Road and buy us all ice cream cones for a nickel apiece, even if it was almost dinnertime.

My mother mixed her first martini at 5 p.m. sharp. The second, a half an hour later. In between, she might pop a tranquilizer. Once the dishes were done, bedtime books were read, and the little kids were tucked away, she'd throw on her nightgown and brush her teeth, then scurry to the side of her bed, where she'd kneel, take a deep breath, and bow her head. After making a quick sign of the cross over her chest, she'd bury her face in her hands. I always wondered what she was praying for so intently. Thanks? More energy? A way out? Only then would she hop under the covers and, with the world's widest shit-eating grin, declare herself, *Just happy to be in bed.* By 8 or 9 p.m., she was down for the count. The house was more or less all ours to do as we pleased.

Holmer tried his best with us, too. He would swoop into the house from New York City on Friday nights, tipsy from airplane booze, and make his way around the kitchen table.

Put your cheeks up here, he'd say, yanking our faces toward his as he kissed us all so hard that we shook like Jell-O. He'd call us his "little tort-feasors," a term he learned in law school that we thought sounded like a German swear word. After another highball or two, he'd lie on the play-room floor and hoist us up on his legs so we could fly like little helicopters, squealing and squiggling. We called them our "dangerous tricks."

Holmer performed all the duties expected of a father with a brood of our size. He helped coach Little League baseball in the spring and foot-ball in the fall and presided as the lector at Sunday mass, winking at us from the pulpit whenever the readings referenced "asses" or "the bosom of Abraham." In later years, after he stopped traveling so much, he served as president of the parish school board, and, for a time, he and my mother taught religious instruction to high school students, exorting them to be like Jesus and treat each other with dignity and respect.

But at home, Holmer was fidgety, Mr. Ants in Your Pants, a constant motion machine, scrubbing the kitchen counter, snapping his fingers, tap-ping his toes. He couldn't keep our names straight. When he was especially flustered, he'd spit them out at once. "MaryNancyJeanGirl." The boys were simply "Dilly," a combination of Danny and Billy.

We made him nervous. Holmer never learned how to cope with a houseful of screaming kids. His mother had hit him. So, he hit us. These were not the controlled spankings once sanctioned by the preeminent pediatricians of the day like Benjamin Spock. They were more spontaneous actions, spasms of his monkey brain—jabs to the ribs, a smack to the side of the head, a punch here and there, a crack from his belt if we were really bad, one from the belt's buckle, if we were really, *really* bad.

What, if anything, were you thinking? he'd scream as he inspected the half-assed job one of us had done sweeping the garage or raking the lawn. *Give me that thing.* Then he'd grab the broom or the rake, hip-check us out of the way like a hockey defenseman, and finish the job himself. By Saturday afternoons, we'd all be tiptoeing around the house, steering well clear of him until he left for New York again on Monday morning. Sundays were the worst, especially if he was hungover and the Chicago Bears had lost another football game. Even the slightest drop of spilled milk could set him off then.

Holmer loved that damn football team. He would sometimes sneak us into Bears games by hiding one of the little ones under his coat or have a few of us whiz past the usher while he pretended to be fumbling for the tickets. But the team disappointed him more often than not. A season ticket holder, he once threatened to sue them for a breach of fiduciary duty, claiming they were only "masquerading as a professional football team" to bilk fans like him out of their hard-earned cash.

When he was in a hurry to get out of the house and we were in the way, Holmer would flail his arms as he hustled toward the front door, sometimes with a mug of scalding-hot coffee in one hand, shouting, *Look out! I'm coming out swinging!*

He often looked ashamed after one of these outbursts, though he'd never say as much. You could see the regret in his eyes, the way he avoided looking right at us.

Here. Try this, he'd say, staring at his feet as he handed one of us a bite

of steak that he was grilling or some other peace offering like a salted rad-
ish or some pickled cucumbers. I'd reach out and take one of his scraps
even if I didn't want it, just to make him feel better, to put an end to the
awkwardness. It scared me to see him lose control like that. Ten minutes
later, he'd be shaking his butt, doing a little dance, singing a silly song:

OH . . . What'll ya have, the waiter said, casually picking his nose.

I don't think he meant to hurt us. He just didn't know how not to.

Our father's sudden mood changes and our mother's melancholia
made us tense, like little deer teetering through the forest, vulnerable and
unprotected. We fretted that the tigers could come bounding toward us
at any second. Or, maybe, they'd creep up on us slowly, slinking through
the glades, as tigers often do.

As we grew older, Patty and I added other rituals to our bedtime repertoire, ones we hoped could steady us a bit. With no parent available to
settle us to sleep, we tried to train each other to shut up, sleep tight, don't
let the bedbugs bite. Just after turning out the lights, Patty and I would
chant:

*Order in the courthouse! Speak, Monkey, speak! The next one to speak
is a monkey for a week. Starting . . . NOW!*

It rarely worked. Patty did well enough, but my lack of impulse control would get the best of me. I'd pretend to be choking or having a sei-
zure, anything to coax her into talking.

You okay? Patty would whisper, earnestly scampering to my rescue.

Monkey! I'd screech.

And our mother would shout out to us again. *Pipe down, you two!*

That would only make us laugh harder. And back we'd go, bouncing
from bed to bed, hooting and squealing as we pretended to be playing
imaginary flutes.

We wanted to be good. We tried our best to be brave. Once, we dared ourselves to fall asleep holding hands over the Tiger Pit. But we never stopped worrying about the beasts that we imagined swirled between our beds. We knew we were no match for them, and we dreaded the day that they would rip us apart. It seemed like only a matter of time.

Indeed, one day, the tigers did come.

THEY WERE NOT REAL tigers, of course, but a menace just as ferocious, with power just as deadly. They scratched and clawed until they made mincemeat of us all. Some in our family were devoured from head to toe, never to be seen again. A sister, ripped to shreds and swallowed whole. Then, years later, a brother, snatched before our very eyes. We could see it happening. We just couldn't do anything to save him. Or maybe we were too scared to try.

Those of us who were left tried to hide. But the beasts were relentless. Just when we thought we were free, one would spring toward us. And then another. And another. Eventually, we were all mauled and mangled. No one escaped unscathed.

In time, we learned that if we were to survive, we couldn't just shiver under our covers the way Patty and I used to. We'd each have to figure out a way to fight back, wrestle those fuckers to the ground, pound them into submission once and for all.

If not, they'd surely come back and get us, too.

2

Get Out of Jail Free

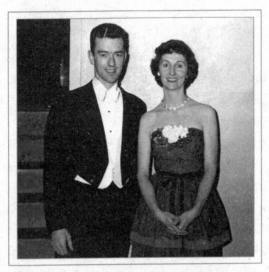

My mother and father going out on the town.
Fox Point, Wisconsin, 1950.

I f my mother had gotten her way, my siblings and I would have never been born.

She was so afraid of what might happen if she married Holmer that she tried to call off their wedding just weeks before the ceremony. *Too late,* her father said as the August 1951 date drew near. The invitations had already been mailed. Besides, he wasn't going to allow her to embarrass the family by doing something so crass.

Don't blame me, my mother would tell us when Holmer exploded in a rage or danced around the breakfast room table in one of Grandma's sequined hats. *I tried getting out while the getting was good.* But we heard them giggling in their bedroom often enough to know how she really felt. Night after night, Holmer chased my mother around the kitchen, pinching her butt, throwing his arms around her waist, and kissing her cheeks. She pretended not to like it, rolling her eyes and pushing him away. But no one bought her little act. I caught them dancing in the living room late one night while Peggy Lee's smoky voice wafted from the hi-fi, promising the best is yet to come. My mother wrapped her arms around my father's neck and sank her head into his chest like she was melting right into him.

She loved playing the straight man in their romantic comedy routine. *Wanna roll?* my mother would ask Holmer as she handed him a basket of bread at dinner. He'd wiggle his eyebrows, lean into her, and whisper, loudly enough for us all to hear: *Think we have time?*

I always assumed that my mother wanted to back out of their engagement because she was nervous about what a nut my father was. "Wild Bill," as he was widely known, was so hyper as a boy that when the Dust Bowl fires stretched all the way to the woods of northern Wisconsin in the early 1930s, he would try to run *toward* the fire wagons. Fearful for his safety, his mother would dress him up like a girl, figuring that he'd be too embarrassed to go outside and be seen in a frilly frock. When that didn't work, she tied him to a tree.

One of the nuns who taught him at St. Robert School in Shorewood, Wisconsin, grew so tired of his shenanigans that she slammed him up against a wall hard enough that the clock hanging above him stopped and never started again. Holmer proudly claimed that the nuns kept the timepiece up there for years as a warning to other children about what could happen to them if they were as incorrigible as Bill Kissinger.

But Holmer's feistiness wasn't the only reason my parents almost didn't get married. My mother also worried about what Holmer would think if he knew the truth about her.

My parents were fixed up on a blind date in the early spring of 1950 by Grandma, my father's mother, of all people. Holmer was in his first year at Marquette University Law School, compliments of the GI Bill. My mother was teaching kindergarten at the Brown Street School in the poorest section of Milwaukee to children with disabilities, many of them the sons and daughters of immigrants with names like George Washington and Christopher Columbus.

Grandma, who fancied herself a skilled matchmaker, spied my mother at St. Monica Catholic Church as she was returning to the pew after receiving Communion one Sunday morning, and the wheels began to turn. She knew about my mother from Bill Dorward, her new son-in-law. His parents played bridge with my mother's parents. Grandma figured that this Jean Gutenkunst would be an excellent catch for her boy. *Nice family,* Bill Dorward confirmed, rubbing his thumb against the side of his index finger. *Lotta this stuff.*

It was true. My mother grew up in Fox Point, one of the more exclusive suburbs of Milwaukee, where her father, Charlie Gutenkunst, was a village trustee. Charlie's father, my great-grandfather, started a foundry on Milwaukee's south side in 1885, where they manufactured tools for harvesting hay and later railroad parts, vises, clamps, wrenches, and braces. The Gutenkunsts were frequently featured in the society pages as one of Milwaukee's most prominent families. They had a summer house on nearby Pine Lake, a Rolls-Royce, and a live-in maid, even during the worst days of the Great Depression. My mother, the oldest, and two of her three brothers attended private schools and took lessons in ballroom dancing, tennis, archery, horseback riding, and golf. Her father served as president of the Wisconsin Club and an officer at both the Town Club and the Milwaukee Country Club.

Holmer's family, by contrast, was always hard up for cash. His father, Matthew Kissinger, one of eight children, dropped out of school after sixth grade to help make ends meet, doing odd jobs, fixing cars, and selling vitamins. Matt was a voracious reader and a hard worker, but he had trouble getting ahead during the Depression. Sometimes, money was so tight that they had to rent out the bedrooms of their Shorewood bungalow while Holmer and his brother and sister slept on cots in the hallway. Christmas 1932, the same year that my mother received a dollhouse with electric lights and running water, Holmer begged for the sailor suit that he had seen in the window at Schuster's department store in downtown Milwaukee.

Oh, we could never afford that, Grandma told him.

But when six-year-old Holmer bounded downstairs on Christmas morning, he discovered the little navy-blue suit with the matching hat and grosgrain ribbon nestled under the tree. He jumped up and down with glee and spent the day marching around the house, fighting imaginary pirates. His joy was short-lived. The next day, Grandma made him fold up the uniform and put it back into the box. Then they hopped on the streetcar and returned it to the store for a full refund. He was crushed.

As Grandma watched my mother walk back from Communion that Sunday, she knew that her boy would be set for life if he could snare the Gutenkunst girl. So, she set the trap with help from a little unexpected inheritance, her portion of the sale of her family's farm. Instead of investing her windfall in the stock market or parking it in a savings account, Grandma bought Holmer a red convertible, hoping that would catch my mother's eye. Holmer, now twenty-three, had jet-black hair, piercing brown eyes, a square jaw, and chiseled looks good enough that he landed top modeling jobs in town. He didn't need his mother's help finding romance. In fact, he already had a girlfriend named Joan. But Grandma was going for the big payday, betting everything she had on the girl with the family fortune.

By anyone's accounting, my mother was quite a prize. A Junior Leaguer with a pilot's license, she spoke French and studied English literature at Carleton College (two of her brothers were Princeton men). Her friends called her Curly—not for her hair (which indeed was curly) but for her toes. She had big, doe eyes, legs that could rival Betty Grable's, and the cutest dimples Bill Kissinger had ever seen. She was quiet—shy even—but get a few martinis into her and she could belt out all the words to "Mimi the College Widow."

My mother secretly worried that Holmer was too much for her. He danced on top of bars, guzzled beer, and introduced her to his friends as Jean "Dirty Word."

It's Guten-KUNST, she'd say, trying to hide her amusement with a scowl of false indignation. *KUNST means "art."*

Holmer nicknamed my mother "Maude," after a foulmouthed old battle-ax who worked the counter at the Milwaukee County Courthouse, where he and his fellow law school students spent hours poring over case files. Holmer made my mother laugh. And she needed a good laugh. Her mother, Chloe, was dying of breast cancer, and the mood at home was grim.

My mother was twenty-four years old and terrified of losing her mother. Chloe was always so breezy and cheerful. Without her, who would remind my mother to be brave, to believe in herself, to know that—no matter what life brings—she must have faith that things will get better?

Chloe died late that November. Now, in the dead of winter, my mother spent her evenings cleaning out her mother's closets and writing thank-you notes to the funeral guests while her father refilled his martini glass and sulked in the corner of the living room, often without even bothering to turn on the lights. Adventures with Holmer in his shiny red convertible offered just the escape my mother craved.

As unlikely a pair as they seemed to be on the surface, my parents would come to discover that they actually had a lot in common. Holmer, it turned out, was not just a party boy in search of an easy payday, and my mother was more than a well-mannered trust fund baby looking to laugh her way out of her grief. They were each stuck in a bad situation, eager for a fresh start. They both longed for someone who knew how it felt to have your life sailing along in one direction and then, suddenly, one day, without any warning, to have it be turned around so completely that you didn't know where you were heading anymore.

Each was haunted by family shame that they tried to drown in gallons of gin. They were jittery deep down inside, worried that they weren't good enough. How could they ever stack up against their A-list debutante / law school crowd? They learned early how to pretend like nothing was wrong. Glide on your charm.

Besides, they had no business complaining. They were the lucky ones, not like their poor brothers, both named John, one who died in August 1943 and the other who was born two months later.

HOLMER'S BROTHER, JOHN MATTHEW Kissinger, known as Jack, died on August 16, 1943, long before my siblings and I were born. Grandma and Grandpa barely spoke about him to us, and neither did Holmer. All we knew was that our uncle Jack had been killed in World War II. Holmer kept a faded photograph of the two of them on his dresser. Jack, who must have been about fourteen when the photo was taken, is sitting astride a motor scooter, wearing a leather jacket and a devilish grin. Holmer, four years younger, is standing behind his brother, sporting a pair of knickers and a double-breasted wool coat, smirking. By the looks on their faces, it seemed like they were up to no good and darn proud of it.

Without much information to go on, I used to make up little stories about what might have happened to this dashing uncle: shot down by the evil Nazis somewhere over Europe or maybe by the Japanese near a little island in the Pacific. Holmer's unwillingness to discuss his dead brother compounded the tragedy in my mind, making it not only sad but a little spooky. *What's the mystery?* We were reminded of this each night as we bowed our heads for the blessing of the meal and recited this eerie little coda: *Eternal rest grant unto him, oh Lord, and let perpetual light shine upon him.*

All we knew of our uncle was that Grandpa had had a heart attack when he heard the news of Jack's death and was too sick to attend his funeral. What really happened, I'd learn more than seventy years later, was much more complicated and even more wrenching.

Jack was in his junior year studying history at St. Norbert College and working as a news announcer at WTAQ Radio in Green Bay, Wisconsin, when he was drafted into the army in March 1943, a month before his twenty-first birthday. He was stationed in Stamford, Texas, training to be a pilot, when he learned that his father had suffered a massive heart attack back home in Milwaukee. Jack and Grandpa had always been close, fishing buddies who'd soldiered through their own war together—enduring Grandma's tirades and physical assaults. Grandma had a fierce temper and was quick to use her wooden spoon to crack some sense into her children, particularly Jack. She'd once beaten him so badly that Grandpa, though short on cash as always, paid for Jack and him to stay in a motel for a time. Relatives said Grandma resented how close Jack was to his father, an intimacy she didn't share, and she let them know it with the back of her hand or that thick wooden spoon.

Even with war raging, Jack managed to get his supervisor to grant him a compassionate leave so he could go back to Milwaukee to say goodbye to his dying father. By the time Jack arrived at the hospital, Grandpa's condition had taken a turn. To everyone's surprise, he had started to improve and was expected to make a full recovery. Jack returned to Texas a few days later, relieved about his father's improving health but scrambling now to make up for lost training time. He needed just fifteen more hours of flying to be promoted but would have to hustle, lest his supervisors flunk him.

"Well, I'm back into the swing of things again, and boy-oh-boy: How they do swing!!" Jack wrote in a letter to his mother's oldest sister a few days after he got back to Texas. "I was practicing solo landings and I did LOUSY!!"

Roughly one-fifth of his class had already been demoted. "It's hell watching these guys wash out," Jack wrote.

He had good reason to fret. Those who couldn't cut it were sent back to the general corps as infantrymen, which almost certainly meant being a part of the ground troops fighting Hitler's troops across Europe or slogging through African deserts or Pacific island jungles. At that point in the war, an average of 220 American soldiers and sailors were dying each day. Jack figured it was better to take his chances in the air, even if the rickety planes were so dangerous that he and his buddies referred to them as the "Flying Coffins."

He knew that if he mastered his flying skills, he might become a commercial pilot someday, and wouldn't that be the life? Trips to Los Angeles, Miami, maybe even Paris. He logged out for the last flight of the night just after 5 p.m.

Mrs. W. W. Young and her young son, Charles, were picking cotton in a nearby field when they noticed a plane sputtering out of control, then nose-diving before hitting the ground at a ninety-degree angle. They ran to the plane to see if they could help. "The pilot was still in the cockpit with his head and right arm hanging over the right side," Mrs. Young would later tell investigators. "I said to him, 'Son, is there anything I can do for you?'"

Jack tried to raise his arm three times and to nod. Mrs. Young sent her son scurrying to a nearby farm to call for help while she waited with Jack. She could hear his breathing grow heavier and more labored. Then he started to cough. By the time help arrived more than twenty minutes later, it was too late. Jack was declared dead at the scene.

Grandpa, who had been sent home from the Milwaukee hospital two days earlier, was visiting in the living room with Grandma and some relatives when the doorbell rang. Two army officers stood in the doorway, one with a telegram in his hand. Neighbors said Grandma shrieked so loudly they could hear her from down the block. Holmer, who'd just finished his junior year of high school, was out drinking beer with friends at the time. When he arrived home later that night, the house was dark. He saw the telegram lying on the dining room table.

CAUSE OF ACCIDENT UNKNOWN STOP
PILOT FATAL STOP

Tipsy from beer, Holmer misinterpreted the telegram and thought that Jack was still alive. He went to bed praying for his big brother's full recovery.

Investigators for the Aircraft Accident Board acknowledged that Jack should have been supervised more closely. His judgment was deficient "due to lack of training and experience required to form sound decisions," army investigators noted. He especially should have been warned about the dangers of flying so low. They promised to do a better job of that with the new recruits. But the army assumed no responsibility for Jack's death. As far as they were concerned, Jack's death was his own damn fault. No one else was found to be complicit or would be made to answer any questions about the crash.

They charged Jack with safety violations. He wasn't around to face the charges, of course, but his family would pay the price.

The army issued gold stars to the parents of soldiers killed in battle—including Grandma's sister, Mame, whose son Bob was shot down in the Pacific on a mission he flew as a favor for a friend. Gold Star families were awarded death benefits. They hung banners from their living room windows and wore pins on their lapels to let the world know that their children had died valiantly fighting for freedom. Grandma and Grandpa got none of that. They were left to absorb their grief with the humiliation that their boy was dead because, well, he screwed up.

Decades later, it would be revealed that Jack was one of nearly fifteen thousand American men who died in flight training during World War II, never having left American soil.

Jack's broken body arrived home in a steel casket. The part of the story my siblings and I always heard about Grandpa being too weak from his heart attack to attend Jack's funeral was true. Grandpa stayed home while Holmer, a few days shy of his seventeenth birthday, ushered Grandma up the aisle at St. Robert Catholic Church as they followed Jack's coffin to the altar.

Nine months later, Holmer enlisted in the navy. Because he was only seventeen years old, he'd need his parents' permission, which they gave without hesitation. Two weeks after his high school graduation, Holmer left for training, hoping to become a pilot, just like his brother. He would finally get a sailor suit that his mother could not return.

MY MOTHER WAS MORTIFIED when she discovered that a baby was on the way. A baby! The year 1943 had already been a hell of a mess. World War II was raging, and even some of her well-heeled male friends were no longer able to get deferments. Watching them go off to war was awful. Then there was the damn car crash. Her sedan slid on some black ice midway through her senior year of high school after a night of heavy drinking at her family's lake house. My mother broke her neck and had to wear a body cast for the remainder of the school year. She ate her meals standing up with a plate propped up on the living room mantel. She missed so much school that she was not allowed to graduate with her class and had to take summer classes to be able to start college on time that September.

Now this. Her mother is *pregnant?*

But what if the neighbors think the baby is mine? she asked her mother.

John Woodward Gutenkunst was born on October 15, 1943, while my mother was away at her first year at Carleton College. The minute she met her newborn brother, my mother knew something was wrong. Johnny's limbs were floppy, and his eyes slanted upward. He had trouble sucking.

Probably best for everyone if you don't even hold him, dearie, the labor and delivery nurse told my mother's mother, Chloe. The hospital would find a good home for him where the nuns could care for him. But Chloe would hear none of it. She took her baby home and cheerfully introduced him to friends and relatives, pretending that nothing was wrong.

Secretly, she was devastated. Chloe felt guilty for having a baby at the age of forty-three. She knew that the older the mother was, the more likely it was that the baby could be born with complications. Her husband, Charlie, my grandfather, had always been a brooder. No one said it out loud, but it was clear to my mother that her father struggled with depression. He would sit in dark rooms at night and go for long stretches without talking, so that even his children were sometimes frightened of him. My mother had heard whispers about how her father had spent some time in a psychiatric hospital before she was born. She worried that the stress of the new baby, with his obvious medical needs, would send her father into a tailspin.

When she was home for Christmas break and again the following summer, my mother tried to tell her parents that Johnny needed special help, but they refused even to discuss it. Precious time was wasting away.

Johnny was not getting the early intervention that could have helped him with his language and motor skills.

It was only after a nanny insisted that Johnny be examined when he was nearly a year old that Chloe and Charlie took their son to see a specialist in Chicago. The doctor took one look at the toddler and delivered the news in no uncertain terms: *This child has mongolism,* now known as Down syndrome. *He won't be able to talk intelligibly or look after himself,* the doctor warned them. *With lots of supervision, he may learn to wipe his bottom and dress himself, but he will never read or write. He may have trouble breathing, and his heart likely will grow weaker each year.* The doctor saved the most heartbreaking news for last. Most "mongoloids," as they were then called, rarely lived past puberty. Nearly half died in the first year.

By then, my mother was back at college. Her diaries discuss her thoughts on Chaucer (*Ugh!*) and Virginia Woolf (*Wow!*), trying to find a date for the spring formal (*Slim pickings*), her latest bowling score (*Don't ask*), and how to mix the perfect Manhattan. No mention was made of her baby brother.

Not long after that, my grandmother Chloe discovered a lump on her breast.

Let's keep an eye on that, the doctor said. *Could just be stress.* It wasn't. By the next year, the cancer had spread to Chloe's organs. When she grew too weak to care for Johnny, Chloe realized she couldn't delay the inevitable any longer.

Reluctantly, she agreed with her husband that it would be best for everyone to send their young son someplace else to live. Johnny had just turned six. My mother had graduated from college and moved home. She was teaching kindergarten for children with special needs and offered to stay home and care for her little brother instead, but her parents said no.

You need your own life, her mother insisted.

The Gutenkunsts certainly had the means to pay for Johnny's care. My grandfather's business was going gangbusters, especially now that the war was over.

They chose to send Johnny to St. Coletta School for Exceptional Children, an institution for children and adults with disabilities run by Sisters of St. Francis of Assisi in Jefferson, Wisconsin, sixty miles from the Gutenkunst home. Heartbroken, Chloe consoled herself with the notion that she was not shipping off her precious little boy to some broken-down human warehouse on the outskirts of town. The tidy campus, with its Georgian Revival buildings made of Cream City brick, featured a chapel, theater, swimming pool, grand piano, and even a small golf course.

The school, begun in 1904 as St. Coletta's Institute for Backward Youth, was in its heyday when Johnny arrived in 1949, hailed as the nation's premier institution for people with disabilities. It was home to 500 residents from all over the country who were cared for by a staff that included 103 nuns. Later that year, Rosemary Kennedy, sister of the future president, came to live there after a lobotomy left her without the ability to talk intelligibly or care for herself. St. Coletta's proved to be a perfect hideaway for her, tucked in between the cornfields, far from the glare of the national media.

The children attended school and church, while the older residents tended the plants in the greenhouse, put on plays, picnics, and pageants, and helped care for the horses, cows, chickens, and pigs that lived in nearby barns. Johnny lost his first tooth there. *Such a cheerful child,* the nuns said. But was he really? It was easier to believe that, my mother knew. If the family pretended like he was happy here, then surely he must be. *Johnny loves singing and dancing,* the nuns said. But Johnny barely spoke a word. They found it especially endearing how he cheered enthusiastically at every football and basketball game, regardless of which team had scored.

Families coming to visit the campus said they found comfort in the familiar words from St. Matthew etched over the transom of the main entry:

INASMUCH AS YE DID IT UNTO ONE OF THESE MY BRETHREN, EVEN THESE LEAST, YE DID IT UNTO ME.

"These least"? Chloe didn't consider her little boy the least of anything, and it pained her not to be able to care for him any longer. Johnny never moved home again. Chloe died of breast cancer eighteen months later at the age of fifty.

BY THE TIME MY parents went out on their first date, they were both eager to put the sadness of their families behind them and plow a new path.

Grandma's gamble had hit pay dirt.

On March 17, 1951, about a year after their first date, my mother and father made a pit stop at Gesu Catholic Church on Marquette's campus for a little prophylactic confession before heading off to the bars. It was St. Patrick's Day, after all, and it was sure to be a bit of a bender. While my mother slipped into the confessional, Holmer reached into his pocket and pulled out the one-carat square-cut diamond ring set in platinum that Grandma had bought for him a few weeks earlier. He wedged it onto the crucifix of his rosary and handed it to my mother as she made her way to the rail to say her penance.

The diamond sparkled as it reflected the stained glass, and my mother stared at it for several minutes, feeling light-headed enough to faint. She waited until saying her Hail Marys before grabbing Holmer's arm and heading toward the door. *Yes,* she said as they stepped into the frosty night air, *I will marry you.* They kissed at the top of the steps, their souls newly wiped clean of sin. Then they made a beeline to meet their friends at the Silver Spring House, a tavern a few miles out of town, where they drank themselves into a stupor.

The wedding was scheduled for the following August. It would be a lavish affair with three hundred guests at St. Monica's Catholic Church in Whitefish Bay, followed by a reception at the Milwaukee Country Club, the society pages of *The Milwaukee Journal* and *Milwaukee Sentinel* announced.

Upon more sober reflection, my mother was not so sure that this was a good idea.

A few weeks before the ceremony, she told Holmer that she needed to let him know something very important. What she was about to say might come as a shock. Still, she wanted him to hear it from her.

He could not imagine what this might be all about. Was she pregnant? If so, the baby certainly was not his. As Catholics, sex before marriage was strictly forbidden, though plenty of people violated that rule. Holmer and my mother, however, did not, tempted as they may have been, or so they always told us.

Pregnant? *No,* she said. *Worse.*

She wanted him to know that the past few years had been very rough as she watched her mother grow sicker. She felt shaky, confused, scared. *I have these spells,* she said, *times when the air feels thick and it is hard even to move.* Then my mother took a big breath and blurted it out: She had seen a psychiatrist. Furthermore, she was taking medication for her dark thoughts. My father was stunned.

He never knew anyone who had been to a psychiatrist or took pills for something like that. Milwaukee, then a city of 650,000, had just one psychiatrist listed in the phone book. If other people had mental problems, they did not discuss them with him. Holmer's mind raced. He wasn't sure what to think.

What if my fog never lifts? she asked him. *Would it be fair to saddle you with this for the rest of our lives?* She wondered, was Holmer really the right one to marry? Maybe someone calmer, steadier, maturer would be a better fit.

This is your Get Out of Jail Free card, she told him. *No one would blame you if you called off the wedding now.* He sat there in a daze, not knowing what to say.

Later that night, she told her father that the wedding was off. She was still too raw from having just lost her mother, and she wanted to wait until she felt stronger before making such a big move. *Absolutely not,* her father said. He wasn't going to let her embarrass him like that. How do you uninvite three hundred people and return all those gifts? Besides, they'd already given a preliminary headcount to the caterer. *You'll be fine,* he told her.

So, she acquiesced, taking her chances that this marriage, beginning on the shakiest of grounds, might somehow turn out all right.

As August 18, 1951, dawned, my mother slipped into her imported

Belgian lace gown with its matching veil. She tucked a handkerchief that belonged to her mother under one sleeve. It was a poor substitute for having Chloe at her side on this momentous day, but this was a little piece of her nonetheless, and it would have to do.

The guests started filling the pews as the organist serenaded them with Vivaldi, Brahms, and then Bach. Grandma, the old matchmaker, beamed as she took it all in from the front row, just a few yards from the spot where she'd first spied my mother streaming back from Communion eighteen months earlier. By 11:00 that morning, the deed was done. Holmer and my mother hoisted crystal champagne goblets and kissed for the camera as the wedding guests cooed and clapped their approval for these adorable newlyweds.

Midway through the reception, they realized that they both had too much to drink. So, Holmer slept it off in the passenger's seat while my mother, who was just slightly less intoxicated, drove the ninety miles to their wedding night suite at a hotel in Madison. The next day, they continued west toward a dude ranch in Colorado. To my mother's dismay, the place was full of single women, teachers in the waning days of their summer vacations. After three nights of watching her new husband square-dance with nearly every one of them, my mother suggested that they finish the honeymoon elsewhere. They headed to Denver and checked into the Brown Palace.

The following week, the newlyweds returned to Fox Point, moving into my mother's childhood home with her newly widowed father just down the hall. Holmer began his second year of law school, and my mother went back to the kindergarten classroom, this time at the Fox Point School, just a few blocks from their home. They tried to be as quiet as two young lovers could be lying in front of the living room fireplace late at night. But no one was surprised when the doctor called a few weeks later to deliver the news: My mother was pregnant.

And so it began. Their darling baby girl Mary Kay was born that June with a shock of thick black hair. Nancy arrived the following year, and a boy the year after that. They named him John Matthew in honor of Holmer's dead brother. He'd later be nicknamed "Jake."

Holmer had graduated from law school by then, but he opted not to enter into a law practice. He'd found that he could rake in much bigger bucks turning on his considerable charm hosting three-martini lunches and selling pharmaceutical advertising than he could pulling all-nighters mapping legal strategy as an associate at even one of the most exclusive white-shoe law firms. "Better living through chemistry," the chemical industry's motto, also meant a better way for Holmer to make his living.

By 1956, my parents had moved to Chicago, where Holmer and his business partner founded *Physicians Management*, a magazine directed toward doctors who owned their own practices. The articles offered investment strategies and tips for running efficient businesses. But the magazine's real value came from the dozens of ads touting the amazing therapeutic values of the new brands of chemical compounds being patented in postwar America. These "miracle drugs" were designed to alleviate "jitters," "executive stomach," and "housewife nerves." More than 35 million prescriptions for the antianxiety drug known as Miltown were sold in the United States in 1957 alone, the equivalent of one prescription per second. That included my mother, who fancied chasing hers with a nightly martini or two. Dashing as ever in one of his dozen or more Brooks Brothers suits, Holmer was cashing in on America's collective anxiety attack.

In February 1957, my mother called her father to wish him well on some throat surgery he was having that day at the Mayo Clinic in Rochester, Minnesota. *It's no big deal,* her father said. *I should be home in a few days.* Conversations with her father were always so strained. *Well, here's some good news that's sure to cheer you up,* she said. *I'm expecting again!* Her fourth baby in five years. Silence.

You're nuts, my grandfather told her shortly before hanging up. The operation was not as harmless as he had let on. Midway through the procedure, he started hemorrhaging on the operating table. Doctors said they tried their best to stop the bleeding, but years of hard drinking had damaged my grandfather's circulatory system. A few minutes later, he was dead at the age of fifty-six.

I was born the following August. Though I never met this mysterious grandfather with his slicked-back hair, dimpled chin, and deep-set brown eyes, I often wondered what he would have thought if he knew that my mother was only halfway through her baby-production operation. Patty came a year and a half after me, then Billy then Danny. By the time Molly arrived, Holmer had grown so weary of driving my mother to the maternity ward, he told her to just take a cab.

3
Secret Hiding Places

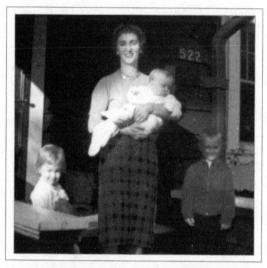

*Me, my mother with Patty, and Jake on the front porch
of our first house in Wilmette, Illinois, 1959.*

Here's the first clue I had that something strange was going on in my family that no one was willing to discuss:

In late July 1963, a few weeks shy of my sixth birthday, I dashed downstairs for breakfast to discover that my mother was gone. No warning. No explanation. She was just gone. I looked everywhere for her.

We had just moved back to Wilmette, a suburb of Chicago, after an eleven-month stint in New Canaan, Connecticut, and our new house was full of unpacked boxes. Maybe she fell into one of the crates with all our winter coats, I thought. I checked the attic, then the basement, then the garage. By lunchtime, I was panicking. No one would tell me where our mother had gone or when she'd be back. She would be back, right?

Get in the car, Holmer barked at me early that afternoon. Patty and I climbed into the back seat of the station wagon with a red vinyl suitcase between us. We had no idea where we were going or why. We watched out the windows as the elm trees lining the street of our new neighborhood morphed into the sororities and fraternities of Northwestern University's campus in Evanston, the jazz clubs and carryout joints of Rogers Park, and then the skyscrapers of downtown Chicago. Patty, who was four years old, growled a little, as she often did when she got nervous.

Cut that out! Holmer snapped from the driver's side as I absentmindedly kicked the back of his seat. I could see his eyes darting back and forth in the mirror as his fingers tapped the steering wheel. The car was hot and sticky, and the afternoon sun was streaming in, hitting me right in the eyes. Holmer weaved in and out of lanes as we rolled down Sheridan Road onto Lake Shore Drive. The jerking motion was making me sick.

We pulled up in front of a brownstone along Chicago's historic Gold Coast. The place looked a little haunted, built from big blocks of sand-colored stone framed by a green turret and a black gate with sharp iron pickets. I grabbed the rail, and we climbed the steep steps. Holmer rang the doorbell. A minute or so later, a chubby man with a bristle of white hair and the roundest face I'd ever seen opened the door and told us to come right in. We followed him as he lumbered down a dark hallway. Even as the summer heat beat down on the city, the inside of the house felt cold and damp and smelled like garlic. Holmer put our suitcase down and made his way to the kitchen.

Should be just a few days, he told the man and his wife, a stern-faced woman with milk-white skin. The sleeves of her faded floral housecoat were too tight around her arms and I could see her slip hanging down in the back. Patty and I didn't know what they were talking about or much of anything about the man who lived in this dank, dark house, except that his name was Jack McIntyre, a.k.a. Jack Mac.

He was one of Holmer's cousins on his mother's side, part of the Lynch clan, a bunch of wrinkled-faced Irish who talked so fast that, beyond "God love ya," we could barely make out a word they were saying.

Jack Mac was not a stranger. He was Billy's godfather. But I'd seen him mostly from a distance at family holidays when we were hustled into the basement to eat pretzels and drink soda. We'd stand around awkwardly, the girls in our party dresses and the boys in suit coats and ties, trying to impress cousins we saw a few times a year by taking turns to see who could burp the loudest.

The "olders," as they called themselves, stayed upstairs in the living room, clutching glasses of Scotch and reminiscing about summers as children spent on their grandparents' farm, or their mother's cabin in the north woods of Wisconsin. They told the same stories so many times that we could shout out the punch lines from the bottom of the stairs in unison. *They're up there talking about the bear again,* my cousin Brian announced, and we all shouted: *J-j-j-j-j-jack! It's a b-b-b-b-bear!*

The little I did know about Jack Mac made me nervous. He was a lawyer who walked with a limp. We heard that he'd busted his leg in a car crash decades earlier. He had a mustache, which very few men did in those days, at least the men we knew. The facial hair was meant to hide a scar on his lip. And there was more. Word was that he'd been married before, to a "showgirl," whatever that meant, and his mother, Grandma's oldest sister, Noreen, had seen to it that the marriage had been annulled.

Limps. Mustaches. Annulments. It all sounded dangerous to me. Now, apparently, Patty and I would be staying with him, his wife, and their teenage son for the foreseeable future.

Put your cheeks up here, Holmer ordered as he leaned down to give Patty and me a quick peck before heading back to the car. The front door clicked shut. The cousin's wife led us down into the basement where we were to change into our bathing suits.

Their son, Johnny, with bright, shiny red cheeks, who was probably about sixteen. He wore a striped T-shirt and shorts and a thick wristwatch that he checked every few minutes, like a spy.

Time for some fresh air. The five of us crossed Lake Shore Drive to Oak Street Beach, squeezing past hordes of sunbathers stretched out on their blankets as little kids darted around like sandpipers. Patty and I splashed a bit in the lake, then took turns burying each other in the sand. I'd barely recovered from the car ride, and now the racket of the beach was making me dizzy.

Transistor radios blaring. Cars whooshing by. Seagulls screeching. Volleyballs thudding as they hit the sand. Where was our mother?

As the sun began to disappear behind the skyscrapers, we headed back to their house where the cousin's wife made Patty and me take a bath. She scrubbed out our bathing suits, muttering something about me "making a BM" in my pants.

That's seaweed. I was mortified.

What are we doing here? Patty whispered to me.

I had no idea.

Where were our brothers and sisters? Where was our mother? She would go away every once in a while. Sometimes, she'd come home with a baby, sometimes not. Maybe she was back in the hospital.

Why were Patty and I the ones who had to leave? What had we done? Holmer nicknamed us "the Pig Sisters" because we (mostly Patty) didn't pick up our clothes as neatly as he liked. Could that have something to do with this? After dinner, Patty and I curled up on the fold-out couch in the living room, dressed in our matching pink polka-dot pajamas, holding on to one another for dear life. Outside, the city buses roared by and the glare from their headlights scratched the walls.

Then, just as mysteriously as we were dropped off, Holmer reappeared and took us back home, back up Lake Shore Drive, past Northwestern University, into Wilmette and past the Baha'i temple, Gillson Park, and the Michigan Shores Club, then down our redbrick street and up our gravel driveway. We scurried into the kitchen, and there stood our mother, casually licking her martini glass.

Hey, kids, she said as though nothing had happened. *How're tricks?*

I have no memory now of how long we'd been gone. A week? A few days?

It didn't matter. We were home. For now. A few days later, I started first grade.

WITH TWO NUNS SUPERVISING ninety-eight first graders, the odds that an adult would take an inventory of our emotional needs were even worse than at home. Those ladies were there to teach us Latin, how to read and write, do simple math, learn the stations of the cross, and make sure no one got too bloodied in the process. We were best served by going along to get along. Don't rock the boat. Behave or be sorry.

Today, an antsy kid like me would probably have an individual education plan and a prescription for Ritalin. Back then, with nearly fifty children in every classroom, the nuns just stuffed the mouth breathers and miscreants in the back of the classroom so they didn't have to deal with us. No one was asking me or anyone else about our feelings.

Not that we'd be inclined to talk about them anyway. Even the kindest nuns looked menacing in their long black woolen habits, shrouded from head to toe with only their faces and hands poking out. They wrapped big, brown rosary beads around their waists that dangled from their hips. The little silver Jesuses on the crucifixes—their tiny heads wrapped in thorns and their wee arms and legs nailed to crosses—swayed as the nuns clomped across the linoleum in thick, black Red Cross shoes, scaring us half to death. Those women must have been boiling in their robes, but they'd learned long ago how to squelch the suffering. Now it was their job to teach us to do the same.

Nuns, unmarried ladies who vowed to live a life of poverty and chastity, were in charge of our academic and spiritual development. Some assumed that responsibility more skillfully and joyfully than others. I knew from the stories that Mary Kay, Nancy, and Jake told at the dinner table that many of the nuns thought nothing of giving you a swift slap to your cheek or punch to your gut. Everyone knew that if Sister Mary David caught you chewing gum in her class, she'd make you smash it into the top of your head so that the only way to get it out was to cut off your hair. Before she quit the convent to marry a priest, Sister Lawrence

Michael specialized in slamming boys up against the blackboard and jabbing their ribs with her elbow.

Their private lives were a mystery to us. They lived together in a Lannon stone house across the playground from school. My friend Terry Byrne, whose brother was a priest, told me that nuns cut their bosoms off before making their final vows.

Our parish school bulged at the height of the baby boom with families of six, seven, eight, and nine children. Sometimes more. We memorized their names the way we did for the rosters of our favorite baseball teams and rattled them off like machine-gun fire: "The O'Connors: KatiePeggy-SuzyJohnnyEunieDortheaBillyMattPetieCarmel." The cluster of big clans formed a tight network that made communication more efficient, like a massive game of Telephone. Our brothers and sisters played with our friends' brothers and sisters. Long before text messages and the internet, the people of St. Francis Xavier Parish could get to the bottom of a story with the precision of the Associated Press. We all knew about the man down the block who kept a secret second family a few towns over and about the time one of the fathers had too much to drink before five o'clock Mass and stood up during Father Maroney's homily to accuse him of being a Communist.

Our school's team name was the Crusaders, fittingly, because the nuns ran the place like a military operation. We were to be orderly. No talking without being called upon. Raise your hand to speak. Stand when Sister calls your name. Fall to the floor on your knees when a priest comes into the room. I got a stomachache worrying about whether I would be able to remember all the rules.

Luckily for me, Sister Mary Assisi, my first-grade teacher, was not a hitter, though she did dabble in a bit of public shaming. Sister made us each a cardboard cutout of a gingerbread man on the top and a wolf on the bottom. Then she pinned them to the bulletin board for all to see. If you misbehaved, she turned your gingerbread man upside down. After the third time, she sent you to the principal, where, God help you, you'd learn to fall in line.

What's this all about, Margaret? said Sister Ann Christine, the principal, the first time I was sent to her office for being chatty. Her shiny cheeks, framed by her veil, shook as she spoke. Would she pull out her paddle and give me a whack? Or would she make me stand in the corner on one foot, holding a pile of books in each hand?

I swallowed hard. Sister leaned down so that her face met mine. She smelled like Dial soap and mothballs. I could feel my heart thumping. *Here it comes.* I squeezed my eyes shut and braced myself for the inevitable.

Nothing.

Instead, she looked squarely into my eyes and said tenderly, *Try to be a better girl, Margaret. Your poor mother's had enough.*

Enough what? She didn't say.

I wasn't about to push my luck and ask her what she meant. That was that.

No whacks, no slaps. No punches or paddles. Somehow, I'd managed to escape her wrath. All because my poor mother had had enough of something that I wasn't privy to. I floated back to the classroom, giddy with relief.

A few days later, my mother went missing again.

I CAME DOWNSTAIRS THAT November morning, ready for school, and, poof! She was gone again—nowhere to be found. This time, Grandma was standing at the stove. The old lady with purple hair leaned on her cane and reached for the salt as she stirred the pot of lumpy Cream of Wheat, her fat arms jiggling. Where was my mother this time? When would she be back?

Holmer's parents would come down from Milwaukee to help take care of us if my mother was especially frazzled. But they often caused more trouble than they were worth. Grandma was nearly paralyzed with arthritis, so aside from bouncing babies on her ample lap and making popcorn after dinner, wiggling her hips, she couldn't help much around the house, and she didn't drive. Apparently, she did once long before she was married, but she ran the car into a ditch and was too frightened to ever get behind the wheel again. She also had asthma, like Patty. To clean out her sinuses,

Grandma would stick the neck of a steaming pot of water up her nostrils as she sat at the kitchen table. That was command central for her in her housecoat, clutching her oversize rosary and barking out orders at us like a drill sergeant. Like the nuns, Grandma believed in running a tight ship.

No slouching!

Don't run around the house in your stocking feet!

She made us memorize prayers and quizzed us on house protocol, some of which sounded redundant to me:

Be honest, truthful, and pure!

Neat, clean, and orderly!

Always say "please," "pardon me," and "thank you."

When it came to safety, Grandma was unequivocal.

If any man tries to touch your privates, kick 'em right in the power plant!

Our fussing drove her crazy. As far as Grandma was concerned, crying was wasted capital that was better spent getting her dead relatives into heaven. She believed in a place called purgatory, a kind of way station between heaven and earth. Only Jesus and the Blessed Virgin Mother got to go straight to heaven when they died, Grandma said. The rest of us would need to simmer a bit. The length of your sentence depended on how well behaved you were while you were alive. But there was a loophole (there's always a loophole): Your earthly relatives could help shave off some of that time in purgatory by offering up their suffering to God on your behalf.

I never fully understood this quid pro quo, but it is best described as "Our pain equals their gain." By Grandma's calculus, suffering was a good thing to be embraced, chips that you could use as barter. So when Mary Kay crawled over some glass and sliced her shin open to the bone, Grandma didn't take her to a doctor to get stitched up. She told her to offer it up to the poor souls in purgatory. Ditto for the time Patty slammed the door on her hand and when I crashed into a tree on my bike and banged up my "private parts" so badly that I had to wear one of my mother's cotton pads between my legs for a few days.

Hark it up now and quit your bellyaching! Grandma would holler at us, grinning a little at the notion that one of her people might just have been accepted into heaven all the sooner for our suffering.

Grandpa wasn't much better company. He was a whiz at household chores, like tightening cabinet doors, and he once built shelving units in the basement for all our clutter. But he couldn't hear very well, and his stories went on way too long. He was a small man with a flat face, high cheekbones, and, rumor had it, eleven toes. He carefully tore each sheet of Kleenex neatly in half any time he needed to blow his nose. For years, we operated under the misconception, advanced by Mary Kay, that Grandpa was part Potawatomi. He had a kind smile and was quick with puns, especially the double entendres that sailed right over our heads:

Eat every piece of meat and pea on your plate!

The man's nuts . . . Grab 'em!

Everyone seemed to love Grandpa, but I once overheard him snarling at Grandma out of the side of his mouth. *Shut up, Alice, or I'll cram this milk bottle down your throat.* That was enough to scare the hell out of me.

I wanted to know where my mother was. *WHERE is my mother?* Why wouldn't anybody tell me?

The nuns will want to know, I told Grandma, hoping that would get her to come clean. She was always sucking up to priests and nuns, having once nearly joined a convent herself.

Grandma, née Alice Lynch, grew up on a farm twenty-seven miles west of Kalamazoo, the youngest daughter in a family of seven children. Her father, John Lynch, had come to America from county Meath, Ireland, in 1879. Alice was a pretty girl, like her sisters, but she was easily flustered, quick to tears, and given to fits of hysteria. She kept a rosary in her pocket at all times, something to calm her nerves, though it did no good. Grandma seemed destined for the convent, but even the nuns had no use for her, volatile as she was.

Except for Margaret, the spinster (my namesake) who became a librarian, Grandma's sisters married and moved on while Grandma stayed on the farm helping her parents cook and clean and tend to the animals—cows, chickens, and two mules named Jack and Jenny. She met my grandfather,

Matthew Kissinger, a traveling salesman from Milwaukee, a few months shy of her thirtieth birthday. Grandpa's first wife had died a few years earlier while giving birth to their first child, a girl named Violet. His parents took care of baby Violet while he traveled for work and searched for a surrogate mother. Grandpa's best friend, a man named Adolf Graner, assured him that Alice, his new wife's sister, would make a suitable stepmother for the child. *She's a real looker, too,* the friend said. *Come with me to Michigan and see for yourself.* Indeed, she was, albeit plump and more than a little zealous in the religion department. At Grandma's insistence, Grandpa, a Lutheran, converted to Catholicism, and they married on June 22, 1921, after just a few weeks of courting. Grandma moved to Milwaukee to care for little Violet. But the child cried so much that they let her go back to live with her grandparents.

If Grandpa had regrets about his new wife, it was too late now to do anything about it. She was pregnant. Jack was born the following April, followed by Patsy two years later, and then my father, who was born two years after that. The blessing of children did nothing to bring my grandparents together, particularly once the Depression hit and money got tighter. Grandpa was away most weeks on business and steered clear on weekends by going fishing in northern Wisconsin or grouse hunting in the western part of the state. By the time my siblings and I were born, Grandma and Grandpa not only slept in separate beds, they stayed on different floors of their house, as far away from one another as they could get.

I imagine Grandpa always missed his little Violet and likely resented Grandma for scaring away the child. Just thinking about that made me miss my own mother.

Will she be home soon? I asked again.

She's back in the hospital, Grandma said.

For what? I asked.

Grandma waved her hand at me like she was swatting a fly.

I want to know what's wrong with my mother, you old witch, I thought.

But the nuns need to know, I protested.

Tell 'em she's got pneumonia, Grandma said.

I wasn't going to fool those nuns. They knew everything.

I bet the whole parish already knew where my mother was. If you asked me, my mother didn't look sick enough to be in any hospital. Her frosted blond hair was always poufed and sprayed and her dark brown eyebrows were neatly plucked. I wouldn't call her pretty in a movie star way. With her long, straight nose and smooth, milky skin, she was more of a classic beauty like the statue of the Blessed Virgin Mary on the altar at church.

With no solid information provided to me, I began to develop my own theories of where my mother was and why she was gone. Holmer had made a lot of money selling ads for *Physicians Management,* the business magazine that he and his partner had started a few years earlier. Magazine sales were soaring so fast, they felt like they had grabbed hold of a rocket. In the summer of 1962, we moved from Wilmette to New Canaan, Connecticut, where Holmer would oversee the New York side of the business while his partner stayed to supervise operations in Chicago. My mother, pregnant for the seventh time, was sad to leave her friends in Chicago, but she had resolved to support her husband as best she could.

"She really didn't want to go," Linda Fischer, one of our old babysitters, told me when I tracked her down years later. "But she didn't have any choice."

In this era of the new frontier, young bucks like Holmer were stepping out of their comfort zones, taking bold chances. Handsome President Jack Kennedy, with his enchanting wife and their two appealing young children, promised to put a man on the moon by the end of the decade. Even the sky was no longer the limit.

My mother had every reason to believe that the move to the East Coast would lead to greater fortune. Few people could light up a room like my father. Charming Billy, quick with a quip, would look into your eyes and make you feel like the rest of the world had just melted away. Everything about him exuded confidence, from the way he talked out of the side of his mouth, like he was letting you in on a secret, to the way he walked, with a swagger, his shoulders thrown back, chest puffed out. The Holmer of that era seemed to all the world like he held the keys to the kingdom in his back pocket, and, if you were lucky, he'd let you in, too. His go-go can-do spirit intoxicated nearly everyone he met, particularly his customers.

My parents rented a pretty country house on a ravine in New Canaan. Norman Cousins, the editor of the *Saturday Review*, lived across the street, and Eileen Heckart, the Academy Award–winning actress, lived down the block. She and my mother had become so chummy that my mother kept a picture of the two of them on her bedroom mirror. We all loved the adventure of frolicking in the woods of Connecticut, climbing the old stone fences and scaling boulders. My mother bought me a little red cape and matching cap, and I would wait for the bus to take me to kindergarten in front of the Silvermine Tavern, a roadhouse built two hundred years earlier to serve Revolutionary War soldiers. We were near enough to New York City that our parents could take us on weekend adventures to the top of the Empire State Building or on the Staten Island ferry to see the Statue of Liberty.

But by early spring, this grand adventure was beginning to lose its luster. Holmer had become convinced that his business partner back in Chicago was cutting him out of his rightful share of the magazine's profits. By July, he quit his job and filed a lawsuit. Now, eleven months after we'd left Wilmette, Holmer was yanking us back there in a hurry. The new school year would be starting soon. With no time to spare, he went house hunting on his own and bought a prairie-style bungalow in Wilmette about a mile from our old neighborhood.

Maybe all this ping-ponging between New York and Chicago was doing my mother in.

MY MOTHER LOVED OUR NEW Wilmette neighborhood, but she hated the house.

The kitchen's too small, and this stucco looks cheap, she sighed when she walked through the front door for the first time. She had been hoping for something grander like the house she'd grown up in, a brick French provincial with a winding staircase and pocket doors.

As far as I was concerned, we were in heaven. Just like at school, the

1200 block of Greenwood Avenue was crawling with kids, most from big Catholic families like ours. The Binders across the street had six kids. The Clohisys on the corner had ten. The Meskills on the other corner had only five kids but made up for it by having a skating rink in the backyard and a blackboard in their basement. Maureen, the youngest, even had her own nun outfit.

We turned cartwheels on our front lawns, played Wiffle ball until the streetlights came on, and then switched to Ghosts in the Graveyard, darting from tree to tree and crouching behind the bushes until our mothers hollered for us to come inside. One neighbor was a pediatrician; another, a surgeon. So, if we fell out of a tree or crashed our bikes, we just hobbled across the street and one or the other of them would patch us up in no time. Frazier Thomas, host of *Garfield Goose and Friends,* a popular kids' television show, lived next door, and his daughter, Kitty, became one of my best friends. Our houses were so close together that I suggested we try to shake hands leaning out of our respective bedroom windows. Living so close to such a celebrity gave me instant cachet with the kids at school.

Frazier Thomas puts ketchup on his scrambled eggs, I announced with great authority on the playground one afternoon. The seeds of my reporting career were already being sown as I learned how to leverage my insider knowledge for playdates.

The mighty elms that lined our redbrick street formed a kind of leafy cathedral ceiling. Many nights, I lay in bed and stared out the window, pretending that the branches were the arms of God holding us tight.

Since my mother had disappeared again, I'd been having trouble sitting still at my desk and cried easily.

If you use up all your tears now, Margaret, you won't have any left for when you really need them, Sister Mary Assisi said. *Better to save them for when a tiger starts chasing you through the jungle.*

Tigers! Sister knew about the tigers. What did she know about my mother? I was starving for answers. Where was my mother? Why did she leave us? When was she coming home? She was coming home again, wasn't she?

No one would say.

Whenever we had trouble, Sister told us to ask our guardian angels for help. Guardian angels, we learned, are invisible little creatures whose sole purpose is to protect us, like a celestial offensive lineman. *Everyone has a guardian angel,* Sister said. *You must leave room in your life and at your desk for yours.* This sounded like crazy talk to me, but I was yearning for anyone to watch over me, so I scooched over to the side of my desk and waited for my guardian angel to appear. *Let's not forget the saints,* Sister said. *They'll protect you, too.*

Saints, we learned, are noble people, now long dead, with marvelous names like Linus, Cletus, Clement, Sixtus, Cornelius, and Cyprian. They knew how to joyfully embrace suffering as a way to share in Jesus's death and resurrection, Sister told us. Suffering was good, Sister said. *When we suffer, we are walking with Christ.*

Because they are so close to God, saints can advocate on our behalf, Sister said. *Pray to them and ask them to whisper into God's ear for what you need.* We were told to thumb through a book of saints and find one that we liked the most. I found that I fancied Saint Thérèse of Lisieux. "The Little Flower," as she was known, was a spitfire of a girl who'd grown up in France in the late 1800s, about the time that Grandma was born. This kid knew how to keep her piehole shut. Even when she developed tuberculosis and started coughing up blood, she simply spit it into her fancy lace handkerchief and hid the evidence under her pillow, never peeking at it, not telling a soul. I started praying to the Little Flower, asking her to help me figure out what was going on with my mother.

Secrets fascinated me. What a thrill to know something that no one else does. You decide whom to tell and when to tell it. I used to spend hours collecting treasures from around the house—feathers, rocks from the beach, doll shoes, or my mother's perfume bottles—and hide them in a wooden box I called my "secret hiding place." Then I'd try to get my brothers and sisters to guess where it was. Even if they said they weren't interested, which was often, I'd tell them anyway. Then I'd start over again.

But secrets also made me nervous. Secrets required discipline, a quality I knew that I sorely lacked.

ON THE FRIDAY BEFORE Thanksgiving, my mother still missing in action, Sister Ann Christine's voice crackled over the loudspeaker. *Terrible news, children.* Someone had shot the president in the head in Dallas.

We dropped to our knees on the cold linoleum and prayed the rosary. Then the nuns sent us home early. With no mother around to fetch us, Mary Kay, Nancy, Jake, and I walked the ten blocks home. The midafternoon temperature was in the sixties, unusually warm for a late November day in Chicago, and storm clouds were gathering in the southwest. I darted from one tree to the next, trying my best not to pee in my pants.

They think the Russians did it, Nancy said. She looked around, like they might be hiding behind the next tree and she was letting us in on a top-secret intelligence briefing. Even at ten years old, Nancy was something of a conspiracy theorist.

When we arrived at the back door, Grandma was parked at the breakfast room table, per usual, listening to the radio and scanning the afternoon newspaper with her magnifying glass in one hand and shiny brown rosary beads in the other.

Jesus, Mary, and Joseph, the old woman cried out as we paraded into the house. She took off her cat-eye glasses and buried her head in her hands, sobbing, *Irish! Catholic!*

As far as Grandma was concerned, the only thing better than being a Catholic was being an Irish Catholic, and, to her great pride, President Kennedy was both.

Are ya Irish? she'd ask any friend who walked through our back door, in her ersatz brogue. Luckily for us, the answer was almost always yes. Our parish directory read like the manifest on the ship that Grandma's father took from Cork to Ellis Island. We had two families of Sullivans, three of Kellys, Callaghans, O'Connors, O'Connells, O'Hallorans, McHughs, McDonnells, Sheehans, Pritchard, Carews, Burn, Burns, and three families of Byrnes. Classes were canceled every March 17, so we could all celebrate St. Patrick's Day in sacred style. While my parents guzzled screwdrivers and Bloody Marys at our uncle Joe's annual bash, we'd ride our bikes past the public school shouting, "SCHOOL SUCKERS!!!"

Oh, indeed you kids are lucky to be Irish, Grandma told us, giving no heed to our German last name or that of our mother. *We Irish have our faith,* Grandma said, *and when you have that, you have all you'll ever need.* She mesmerized us with tales of Irish martyrs who'd sooner be burned at the stake than renounce their devotion to Christ. I beamed with pride hearing about my fearless forebears who were willing to have their fingernails ripped off, be split in two by horses, or made to poke out their own eyeballs before they'd turn their backs on the Lord Jesus or his holy church. I hoped someday I'd get my turn to be put to the test like that. Surely, this new dead president was now a martyr, too. I could start praying to him for strength while my mother was gone.

We squeezed together on the living room couch in front of the TV a few days later to watch the president's funeral. A team of horses pulled a big wooden box as a little boy in short pants, the one Billy's age, stepped out in front of his mother and gave a salute.

The following Thursday was Thanksgiving, and Nancy announced at breakfast that our mother would be coming home later that day, if only temporarily. This was wonderful news. I still had no idea what had landed my mother in the hospital again, and it was looking like I never would. But there were hints. I knew if I listened hard enough and looked for clues, I might be able to figure this out once and for all.

We were nervous wrecks that day waiting for our mother to arrive. Holmer shampooed the living room rug while Patty and I passed the time playing Barbies, using our mother's ashtrays as bathtubs and making tiny towels out of pieces of toilet paper. Grandpa roasted the turkey while Grandma peeled potatoes or, as she called them in her fake Irish accent, "ba-daydas." At around 3:30 that afternoon, just as the sky was turning purple, we heard the driveway gravel pop, a sure sign that someone was close. We scrambled to the bedroom window and smushed our faces into the cold glass for a better look.

It's her! Patty gasped, and once again, I could hear her wheezing like some-one had sewn a tiny harmonica inside her four-year-old chest. We stood on tiptoes for a fuller view. Patty's heavy breathing fogged the glass, so I gave it a good lick. The sharp taste of the cleaning solution made my tongue sting and my eyes water.

Sure enough, there was our mother, a little wobbly from the looks of it, holding Holmer's arm and making her way up the stone path toward our front door.

I zoomed down the stairs, resolved to be good. I still didn't know where our mother had been or how long she'd be home, but I worried that if I misbehaved, she might leave again and never come back.

I'm trying to re-create the scene of what happened next, but my mind is a jumble of tiny snippets from so long ago. I remember little pieces that don't fit together in a tidy narrative. I recall my mother plopping down next to the fireplace in one of the blue velveteen living room chairs, sip-ping a drink, and fidgeting with her hem. She didn't really look at us, and we were not to stare at her. Nor were we to jump on her or ask too many questions. I remember Jake and me sitting at the dining room table mak-ing finger puppets out of the canned pitted black olives that were only served on special occasions like this.

A good day to you, sir, I imagine myself saying, bowing my index finger toward Jake, stealing little glances at my mother when I could.

Nancy is playing "Für Elise" on the piano while Patty and Billy prac-tice their somersaults in the corner. Mary Kay is feeding Danny, who is throwing scraps from his high chair to the delight of Sam, "the damn cat," as we all called him.

While Grandpa carves the turkey, Grandma peers out from her magni-fying glass and mutters something about how lucky we all were. *There are children in India with nothing to eat,* I recall her saying. *You children don't know how good you have it.*

Grandpa shakes his head. *Shut up, Alice,* he says, jabbing the carving knife into the turkey's thigh.

With that, dinner is served.

This next part is a lot clearer in my mind. We gathered in the dining room, and I wiggled into the chair next to my mother, feeling very proud to have scored a spot next to her.

As it turned out, the mystery of my mother's whereabouts would not be solved that night or for many years to come. It would be the first of many secrets I remember keeping over the years—or trying to keep, making me nervous, flustered.

I didn't even get a first bite of turkey before I was banished from the table. Nancy, who sat across from me and had been sticking her tongue out at me all day, kicked me under the table, and I let out a bloodcurdling scream. That got Danny squawking in his high chair. Holmer jumped up from his seat at the head of the table and grabbed me by the collar. He dragged me up the stairs to my room, growling and grunting with every step. It all happened so fast, a flurry of arms and legs.

My mother was finally home, and he wasn't about to let any of us screw this up. Holmer threw me into the room like I was a rag doll and slammed the door. I lay there, sobbing as loudly as I could, hoping my mother would come to save me. I imagined her opening the door slowly, poking her head in first to see if I was okay. I'd run to her, and she would hug me. Then she'd smooth my hair and tell me it was all right for me to go back downstairs and sit next to her and finish dinner. *We've got pumpkin pie with whipped cream,* she'd say.

But she never came.

No one did.

My thoughts began to race. What if I died? They'd be sorry then. I could see them all gathered around the casket. I'd be lying in the box in my blue St. Francis jumper with the school crest on the left side.

We shouldn't have been so mean to her, Holmer would sob. But it would be too late. I would already be dead.

I can't remember now how long I howled before I finally fell asleep that night. An hour, maybe more. Almost certainly I woke up and got into my pajamas, but I have no memory of that now. In the story I've created for myself of that night so many years ago, the next thing I recall is waking and finding the whole house dark. I remember Patty in her bed next to mine. Danny, the baby, was snuggled in the crib in the corner of our room in his light-yellow Dr. Denton pajamas zipped up tight, lying on his belly with his face to the side and his little butt in the air. My throat was sore, and my head was throbbing. I stumbled down the hallway, running my arm along the wall to guide me. I remember hearing Grandma snore in the next room while her false teeth soaked in a glass on the bathroom sink. Or do I? This sounds like a cartoon. These flourishes are a little too tidy. It can't really have happened that way. But, as I strain to fill in the blanks, that's the way I remember it.

Mom, I whispered. *Mommmmmmmmmm.*

The room glowed with the light from their TV, which emitted no sound, at least none that I can recall. I spotted Holmer lying on his side, smiling slightly and hugging his pillow like he was spooning with my mother. I sidled around to her side of the bed, hoping to burrow in next to her. We all loved to curl there with my mother at bedtime as she read us our favorite books, *Nappy the Dog* and, my favorite, Dr. Seuss's *Happy Birthday to You!*

If you'd never been born, you might be wasn't. A wasn't has no fun at all. No, he doesn't.

I'd often wander into my parents' bedroom late at night after the others were asleep. I'd hop in on my mother's side of the bed to rest my head on her soft, warm belly. Then I'd run my fingers up her arm and feel her scratchy armpit, like sandpaper or the cat's tongue. She'd bat my arm away and roll over with her back to me.

Cut that out, kid, she'd say dreamily.

But the sheet on her side of the bed was cold. I reached for her pillow and tried to smell my way to her—some hairspray, a little whiff of Chanel No. 5 perhaps. Nothing. Just Holmer's tang, a mixture of Old Spice, cigarettes, and bourbon. Or was it rum? I can't recall, but this much I know with dead certainty: My mother wasn't there.

I remember stumbling back to my bed thinking I'd really blown it this time. Why did I have to go and ruin everything by screaming at the dinner table like that? Sister Mary Assisi says, *Try to be a better girl, Margaret. Be more like the Little Flower. She coughed up blood, but no one heard her making a big fuss about it.* She knew how to offer up her suffering to the poor souls in purgatory. She knew how to keep a secret.

4

Dangerous Tricks

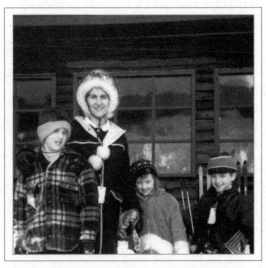

*Billy, my mother, Molly, and Danny on one of our
annual ski trips to the Porcupine Mountains in the
Upper Peninsula of Michigan, 1968.*

I can't say exactly when my mother was released from the psychiatric ward after that Thanksgiving. Her medical records were destroyed years ago, and it's been too long for any of us to remember the specifics. But I do know this: My mother did more than just eat pumpkin pie during her three-hour pass at home that night. Molly, the baby of our family, was born nine months later, almost to the day. Once my mother came home from the maternity ward that August, she stayed put more or less for the next fifteen years, except to go on an occasional spiritual retreat with some ladies from our parish or her annual romantic getaway with Holmer.

Though her mysterious disappearing acts stopped, she now seemed to be encased in a kind of invisible bubble, one that kept us at a distance from her. We didn't doubt that she loved us. She organized birthday parties for us all, baked us angel food cakes, came to most of our basketball games, sewed matching suede jumpers for Patty and me, and decorated our room with lavender and powder-blue daisy wallpaper.

But there was an aloofness about her now, an intimacy that she wouldn't—or couldn't—give us. The medications she took kept her from us. She tuned us out in tiny ways, making half-hearted efforts at scratching our backs or rubbing our feet. My mother had never been one to cuddle or lavish us with kisses the way Holmer often did. When we skinned our knees or a friend said something that hurt our feelings, she'd pat us on the back softly and offer a faint, "There, there." My mother rarely raised her voice. Even her vivid threats of first-degree child abuse—*Come here so I can crack your skulls wide open*—sounded more like a Shakespeare sonnet coming from her singsong voice. We once had a contest at the dining room table to see who could make the meanest, most menacing face. The scariest she could muster was to squint her eyes and pucker her lips slightly like she'd just bit into a lemon.

She didn't dish out words of wisdom or unsolicited advice the way so many mothers did. Nor did she tear up at the kind of events that could cause other mothers to blubber—baby teeth lost, Mother's Day poems scratched in crayon, little girls in white dresses and veils nervously approaching the altar for their First Holy Communion. My mother's feelings were mostly a mystery to us. She rarely talked about her childhood. If you wanted information, you'd have to pry it out of her, pester her with questions. Even then, she might not give much of an answer.

Her parenting approach, like that of many mothers of her generation, could best be described as laissez-faire. She thought nothing of leaving us alone in the toy department at Marshall Field's in downtown Chicago while she and her friends did their Christmas shopping. Once, when I was about six, on a trip to the Brookfield Zoo, my mother loaded me up with so much Dramamine to keep me from getting carsick that I was too drowsy to walk. So, she draped me under a tree and left me there while she and the other kids toured the park. Today, this would be considered felony abandonment. Back then, it was the law of the herd: Do what you can for the greatest number and leave the rest. My mother couldn't be the source of all our emotional nourishment. It wasn't possible. There were too many of us. We'd have to look to each other or elsewhere for that. So, we roamed in packs, taking our chances, oblivious to the danger that lurked everywhere.

We never wore bike helmets or seat belts. No one I knew did. We never owned a car seat. Babies rode in wicker baskets. My mother merely stuck out her right arm when she hit the brakes suddenly to keep one or more of us from crashing into the dashboard or flying through the windshield. For birthday parties, my mother and her friends would hire a man to pick us up in a rusty decommissioned fire engine and transport us to an amusement park in Skokie called Fun Fair. We'd hang over the side of the truck as it weaved its way through city traffic, and climb the ladder for a better view. Inside the park, we'd scramble on rides like the Little Dipper, the Tilt-A-Whirl, and the Wild Mouse, which proved a little too wild once and veered off the tracks.

To the uninitiated, my mother appeared unflappable. She once stood smoking her cigarette and listening to her friend's story in rapt attention at the grocery store entrance, never breaking eye contact, while five-year-old Billy toppled a tower of tin cans a few aisles away. Her friends admired her for how calm and collected she appeared, even as we made a ruckus. But, as we grew older, we became aware that her seemingly cool demeanor was really the result of medication that blunted her natural inclination to anxiety. The truth is, she was often frantic inside. We heard her pacing the hallways at night, humming to herself. We saw her rubbing her thumb nervously back and forth on her chin. The older we got, the more the responsibility for supervising all of us seemed to overwhelm her. She calculated the odds and considered that they were not in her favor. Too many opportunities for disaster: Light sockets. Sharp scissors. Swimming pools. Hyper kids darting around in busy parking lots.

My mother began viewing us with increasing dread, as if sensing that something awful was heading our way and there wasn't a damn thing she could do to stop it. In time, we each gave her plenty of reasons to despair.

Mary Kay flipped the convertible one May morning on her way to class during her junior year of high school. Despite a false report broadcast over the school's public address system that she'd been killed, Mary Kay was saved, she claims, by not wearing a seat belt. She was back in class the next day.

Nancy fell out of a second-story window when she was a toddler and somehow landed in the bushes, seemingly no worse for wear.

On our way home from one of our ski trips in northern Michigan, my parents miscounted as we scrambled back into the station wagon and accidentally left Jake at the gas station. We were miles down the road before anyone realized he was missing.

Uncle Johnny sat on Patty in Lake Michigan during a game of Marco Polo one summer day. We pulled him off her in the nick of time. Patty's curly little head popped out of the water like a jack-in-the-box as she gasped for air.

During the great blizzard of '67, Danny, who had just turned four, attempted to cross the street to play with one of the Clohisy boys and got stuck in a snowdrift up to his neck. We found him, face to the sky, like a bird in a nest waiting for a worm.

When she was two years old, Molly was crawling on the kitchen counter and mistook a bottle of St. Joseph's Aspirin for Children for candy. Childproof caps had yet to be invented, so she easily screwed off the top and ate every one of the orange-flavored tablets. Even after getting her stomach pumped, Molly liked the taste of that medicine so much that she did the same thing a few weeks later.

Some nights, we'd sit around the dinner table gleefully recalling our near-death experiences, competing for the prize of who came closest to actually being killed. I declared myself the champion, by virtue of having slipped into the freezing lake in front of our cousin's cabin in the woods of northern Wisconsin when I was not yet two years old. Jake had been assigned to supervise me, though he was only four, while my parents were busy with baby Patty and the two older girls. The two of us toddled down to the pier, and I fell in. Jake lunged for me, but I floated away. A minute or two later, my body popped up at the end of the pier, facedown, bobbing like a Styrofoam cup. Jake trudged up the hill, sobbing, convinced that I was a goner. He refused to shut up even when my mother scolded him for waking the baby.

But Meggy's lying in the lake, Jake cried.

My mother screamed, and Holmer bolted out of the cabin and bounded down the steps three at a time. He had a recurring dream for decades that he tripped on the stairs and got to the lake a second too late, yanking my icy little corpse from the reeds. As it happened, he dived in, grabbed me by the scruff of the neck, then revived me with mouth-to-mouth resuscitation. My mother wrapped me in a pink wool blanket, plopped me onto her lap, and gave me a few sips of her bourbon to stop my teeth from chattering.

But, when it came to death-defying stunts, no one could hold a candle to Billy. That kid was in a class by himself.

Billy was what Holmer called a "ranger." Even at four years old, he could cover an amazing amount of ground. My mother got a phone call one afternoon from Steve, the family barber, saying that he caught Billy toddling past his shop on Green Bay Road, about a mile from our house. *Can you please come by and fetch the little fella so he can get home safely?* Somehow, Billy's chubby little legs had carried him over the railroad tracks and across a busy state highway. A regular Houdini, Billy could escape anything, it seemed. He was so rambunctious, one of our babysitters refused to take him outside unless she could put him on a leash.

OUR NEW HOUSE WAS just a few blocks from Lake Michigan, close enough that with wind from the east, we could smell the stacks of rotting alewives and hear the screeching of ring-billed gulls as they circled the shore each morning in search of a good meal. My mother would pack the station wagon with towels and suntan lotion and pails and shovels and take us all

to the Wilmette beach nearly every sunny day in the summer. The soles
of our bare feet sizzled as we scurried across the frying pan pavement and
onto the scorching sand. We streamed toward the blue-green water, where
we'd play for hours, pretending to be sharks, bumping butts in games of
Underwater Tea Party or lying on the shore and letting the waves crash
over us, filling our bathing suits with sand.

My mother never went swimming. She didn't want to ruin her hairdo.
No heat or humidity was high enough to risk ruining her hairdresser's
handiwork. She would sooner suffer a little heat stroke than lay all that
to waste.

Each Friday afternoon, no matter what was going on at home, my
mother escaped to the beauty parlor where Jerry, her hairdresser, would
wash, cut, curl, tease, shape, and spray her hair into a furry little helmet.
It was a ritual as sacred to my mother as anything on the altar at church.
For two precious hours each week, she was the one being cared for.

If Patty and I had been good that week, my mother would let us tag
along while Mary Kay or Nancy tended to the littlest kids at home. We'd
spin around in the chairs, pretending we were riding on the teacups at
Disneyland. Or we'd stick our heads under the dryers, imagining that they
were Martian helmets, as we gulped bottles of cold Coca-Cola that we
bought for a dime each from the coffin-shaped machine in the corner. As
Patty and I ran amok around the parlor, our mother closed her eyes and
seemed to float off into space.

As much fun as we had at the beauty parlor, nothing topped the Wilmette beach for adventure, bouncing in the waves, flirting with the un-
dertow. If the sun was a real scorcher, my mother would tiptoe out into
water up to her thighs, scoop a handful to sprinkle on her shoulders, and
let out a little "Whoop!" Mostly, she and her friends would stand like a
pat of flamingos in water up to their knees gossiping and smoking cigarettes, occasionally glancing out at us long enough to take attendance.
Sometimes, they didn't even do that.

One blistering day, Billy went missing. Again. We fanned out in our
usual formation, looking up and down the beach, checking every towel

for our little brother, scouring each bobbing head as the waves of Lake Michigan lapped the shore.

When Billy failed to reappear after we'd searched the beach two times, the head lifeguard blew his whistle and ordered everyone out of the lake. *NOW!*

We huddled by the water's edge as the lifeguards locked arms, forming a human chain. Then they began the ghastly task of combing the water for Billy's lifeless body. I hugged my waist and stared at the waves washing over my toes, trying not to notice everyone looking at all of us. *Where are you, little guy? Please don't be dead.* We tried not to have favorites, but it was clear that everyone loved Billy, with his big brown eyes, raspy voice, and the way he cocked his head to the side like a puppy.

Just then, a woman's voice sputtered onto the public announcement system:

We have a little boy named Michael here at the snack bar who can't find his family. He's wearing red-and-white-striped trunks.

My mother, balancing baby Molly on her hip, flicked her cigarette into the sand and headed toward the snack bar, and we all followed her in single file. Sure enough, there was Billy sitting on the counter, chewing on some Good & Plenty candy. Someone had found him wandering around the locker room, and when they asked him his name, he didn't hesitate: *Michael,* the name of a kid across the street whom Billy admired. *Nice try, kid,* my mother told Billy, and then grabbed his pudgy little hand, yanking him to the ground.

We'd done it again. Somehow, we'd managed to survive with all of us present and accounted for. The day was coming soon enough, though, when such a simple rescue would not be possible.

5
It's All in Her Head

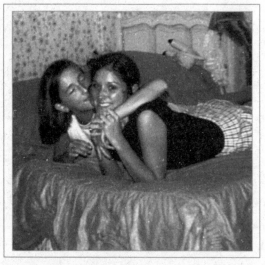

*My legs dangling into the Tiger Pit, I couldn't resist
the urge to give Nancy a little smooch.*

Even now that my mother was home all the time, getting a private
audience with her was next to impossible. If I was going to find a
way to be alone with her, I'd need to employ any means possible.
My big break came when I was in fourth grade, and I got a paper cut in
my left eye so deep that I had to see an eye specialist. He prescribed some
ointment and an eye patch and instructed my mother to bring me back
in a few weeks.

Some kids might have been embarrassed to wear a black eye patch.
Not me. I loved it. Anything for a little easy attention. I wasn't the smartest or the prettiest or the most athletic kid in my class, but I was the only

one with an eye patch that year. I'd seen how medical equipment of any kind—crutches, slings, back braces—could elicit a bit of sympathy, even from the nuns. The year before, I'd taken to wearing Nancy's old, pink eyeglasses to school, hoping they'd afford me a little more gravitas.

Margaret would do a lot better in school if she wore her glasses regularly, Sister Mary David told my mother at the parent-teacher conference that spring. This was the same semester that I got mostly Ds on my report card. Terrified of how these grades would be received at home, I had changed them to look like Bs with my fountain pen.

I think Bs are pretty good grades for her, my mother said as she showed Sister the report card. The old nun, with the jowls of a bulldog, leaned in for a closer inspection and spotted the forgery immediately. She took out her own fountain pen and, with my mother standing there sheepishly, changed the grades back to Ds.

So humiliating, my mother said to me when she got home. *And quit wearing your sister's glasses.*

But this paper cut was the real deal.

On the day of my follow-up exam, my mother picked me up at school in her wood-paneled station wagon, and when I opened the door, I was amazed to see that it was just the two of us. No babies. No dog. Just my mom and me. The radio was on, so we drove in near silence for the fifteen minutes that it took for us to get to the doctor's office in downtown Evanston. I felt very grown-up being allowed to push the elevator button. The doctor leaned toward me and shined a penlight in my eyes. *Looks good,* he said. *No need for further treatment.*

Oh, good, I said, smiling slightly as I slid off the chair. Secretly, I was crushed. What would I do for attention now? We headed toward the elevator. Then something strange happened once we reached the lobby. Instead of heading straight back to the car, my mother took a left and ducked into the diner next door.

Time for lunch, she said. My heart was pounding. Lunch? Here? In a restaurant? My parents went out for dinner nearly every Friday night when Holmer returned from his weekly business trips, but we kids rarely got to go. There were too many of us. We usually stayed home with a babysitter, eating Mrs. Paul's fish sticks and french fries that my mother would cook in her deep fryer, the chunks of ice popping as they hit the boiling grease.

Inside the diner, I felt like Dorothy wandering the land of Oz. So many new sights and sounds and smells. A fan whirred overhead, blowing the aroma of cherry pie. My mother and I settled into a booth next to the counter, where the waitress gave us each a glass of water and a laminated menu with a thick red leather jacket. I ordered a roast beef sandwich and a Green River, a bright lime-green soda popular in Chicago in those days. I can't remember what my mother had, likely a BLT, her favorite.

All those kids back at school are probably doing arithmetic right now, I thought. *Or maybe they are on to reading.* In class, we each took turns reading out loud, trying not to laugh as the boy with the stutter pounded his thigh to steady himself so he could spit out the words. If I were there, I'd be sitting in the back of the classroom, where all the fidgety kids went, boys mostly, who jabbed me with protractors and dared me to eat Elmer's glue. *Like this?* I'd say as I peeled the dried layers of milky white goo off my palm like a sheath of skin after a day of too much sun.

With all the ear infections I'd had as a baby, I usually couldn't hear the teacher anyway. So while the rest of the class studied Nebuchadnezzar and long division, I passed the time by staring at the clock, holding my breath to see how long I could go before passing out.

I wished I could sit still like the other kids. I seemed to be wired differently. When I was especially antsy, Sister Mary David would make me squat next to her at the front of the classroom with my feet in the middle of her enormous army-green metal wastepaper basket and my butt teetering on the sharp rim. It was all I could do to not tip over and spill onto the floor with the rest of the trash in that can. Her metaphor was not lost on me.

Is your bottom good and blistered yet, Margaret? the old nun croaked. I flushed with horror that she was discussing my bottom in front of the whole class, especially the boys.

But I'm not at school now, I told myself giddily. *I'm sitting in a diner with my mother like somebody special, slurping soda through a paper straw.* When my drink was done, I folded the straw in two and stuffed it between my top lip and upper teeth to make walrus fangs. *Oh, Meg,* my mother said and shook her head, chuckling. *What a wag you are.*

And then she looked at me for what seemed like a very long time and smiled so that I could see her dimples. She looked so pretty when she smiled like that.

When we were done with our meal, in no hurry at all, we walked down Chicago Avenue, just the two of us, peeking into a dress shop. I reached for my mother's hand. We moseyed past an antique store with shelves of thick leather books, a big velvet chair, and an umbrella stand. The bookstore on the corner sold purple sweatshirts and wall posters for the Northwestern University students who lived in the dorms nearby.

We didn't talk about anything special. We didn't need to. I watched my mother lean down and look into the windows, and I noticed how glamorous she was with her tangerine lipstick and tweed coat. She smelled like roses.

Okay, kid, she said after a bit. *Back we go.*

I didn't tell anyone about the roast beef sandwich or our window shopping. That was my private time. Mine and my mother's. That night, it was back to business as usual. A stack of dishes for her to clean, baskets of laundry to fold, Billy and Danny and Molly burrowing into her belly as she read them *Nappy the Dog.*

An hour later, long after we were supposed to be asleep, Patty and I were back to jumping over the Tiger Pit, hooting.

Come in here so I can crack your skulls together, my mother called out from her room weakly.

No more Green Rivers or elevator buttons or diners that smelled like cherry pie. Just *shut up and go to bed.* Something inside me ached. I wanted private time with my mother again. I wanted to make walrus teeth out of paper straws to make her laugh. I wanted to see those dimples.

A few days later, I locked myself in the bathroom with a pile of fresh lined school paper. To make sure the edges were good and sharp, I ran my fingers along the side and felt a little sting. A tiny drop of blood began to pool. But that was just a dress rehearsal. *You can do this,* I told myself as I took a deep breath and raised the paper toward my eye.

But no matter how many times I tried, I couldn't slice my darn eyeball again.

Not long after my eye patch came off, Nancy swallowed a whole bottle's worth of aspirin, saying she wanted to die. Then she did it again a few months later. She was in eighth grade and starting to get into trouble at school, ditching class, drinking gin that she would sneak out of the house in glass peanut butter jars, and smoking cigarettes in Gillson Park. One Saturday afternoon, Nancy was arrested for shoplifting a tube of lip gloss at the Montgomery Ward department store in Old Orchard Shopping Center. Now this. Was she really trying to die or just faking it to get out of trouble?

My parents took her to see my mother's psychiatrist up in Lake Forest. Grandma thought that was about the stupidest thing she'd ever heard. *There's nothing really wrong with that girl,* Grandma declared from her breakfast room perch. *It's all in her head.* I was inclined to agree. After all, I wasn't really trying to hurt myself by cutting my eye.

We all faked being sick at one time or another to get more attention or wiggle out of having to go to school. Some dupes were easy to spot. When he was in second grade, Danny declared that he needed to stay home because he had menstrual cramps. Nancy's little pill-swallowing routine looked like nothing more than a little histrionics to me.

A FUNGAL INFECTION THAT killed many of the stately elms of Europe made its way across the Atlantic Ocean in the late 1920s and began spreading west at about the time that we were growing up. By the early 1970s, Dutch elm disease had ravaged the forest cover of Chicago and would go on to claim more than forty million trees nationwide. Day after day, crews of tree cutters would rumble down our redbrick street with their chain saws. The motors growled and sawdust flew as they ripped holes in the sky. Before long, the leafy cathedral that framed Greenwood

Avenue was destroyed. The sun beat down during the day, singeing our Wiffle ball field. At night, the streetlights, once filtered by branches of elms, now glared through the panes with a harshness that made me feel uneasy and exposed. I'd lie at the foot of my bed and stare out the window, squinting as though someone were shining a flashlight right at me, trying to coax some kind of confession out of me.

People began disappearing, too. A teenage boy across the street ran away from home after getting into a fight with his father. I'd look out my bedroom window toward his house and wonder where he was sleeping that night. How did he find food to eat? Several weeks later, we heard he was in California trying to break into show business and that he almost got picked for the role of Robin in the TV show *Batman*.

After a lady down the block suffered her fifth miscarriage, she checked into a mental institution somewhere on the East Coast, and we never saw her again. No explanation. She was just gone, the way my mother had sometimes disappeared years earlier. We kept waiting for her to return, but she never did. The youngest two of her four children would come to our house for dinner every once in a while, and my mother would sometimes take them shopping to buy new clothes.

Eventually, the woman and her husband divorced, and he married his secretary. But for years, the woman and my mother would talk on the phone on Sunday afternoons when the telephone rates were lowest. Sometimes, I stood outside my parents' bedroom door and listened, fascinated by their friendship. They'd formed a kind of secret sorority, stronger, more intense than the crew at the beach discussing winter vacation spots and where to get the best leg of lamb, though there was some of that light banter. My mother would fill her in on news of the block: romantic misadventures of the spinster sisters who lived across the street, decorating updates, the medical reports of various kids' broken bones and burst appendixes.

But then my mother's tone would soften, and there would be long silences while the woman talked. *Yes, I know,* my mother would say in her most comforting voice. *Oh, yes. I know.*

There were other unexplained absences. A high school girl on the next block left suddenly to live with her aunt in Texas. She came home several months later looking puffy and sad. Years later, I learned she'd had a baby that she gave up for adoption.

The odd man who lived a few doors down with his elderly blind mother would disappear and reappear mysteriously, too. We never knew why he still lived at home. *Steer clear of that guy,* Holmer used to warn my brothers. Sure enough, years later, the man was convicted of having sex with underage boys on a boat that he kept at the Wilmette harbor, called *The Slow Poke.*

The world beyond Greenwood Avenue seemed equally harsh and un-forgiving. Each week, the mailman delivered our copies of *Time* and *Newsweek* magazines with increasingly gruesome photos: bleeding U.S. soldiers trudging through rice paddies, Vietcong bodies stacked up like cordwood, sobbing children, one naked, her mouth wide open as she ran down the road to escape the napalm bomb that destroyed her village. The evening newscasts showed daily tallies of soldiers killed.

Not all the casualties were on foreign soil or even part of the official count. Michael, the boy that Billy claimed to be that day at the beach, had an older sister whose husband came home from Vietnam addicted to heroin. A few years later, they found him dead in a gas station bathroom on the west side of Chicago.

On an early spring afternoon in April 1968, my friend's older brother stood off to the side watching us play basketball. *Did you girls hear the news?* he asked. The night before, civil rights leader Martin Luther King Jr. had been gunned down on a motel balcony in Memphis. The older brother spit and turned away, muttering, *The only good King is a dead King.* The harshness of his words made my throat close and my eyes sting, not that I hadn't heard racist language before, especially on the playground of our lily-white Catholic school, where it seemed easy to belittle anyone who didn't look like us.

Two months later, we woke up to the news that Bobby Kennedy had been assassinated as he made his way through a hotel kitchen after winning the California Democratic primary. Mary Kay had been out that night at a baby shower for one of her friends, who was pregnant at fifteen. The hard realities of life seemed to be catching up with everyone.

Late that August, on the first night of the Democratic National Convention, I was sprawled on the family room couch with my mother, watching the local news. The convention was only about eighteen miles from our house, not far from where Patty and I had stayed with Holmer's cousin Jack Mac and his family. Protesters had gathered outside the hall, demanding an end to the Vietnam War. Mayor Daley was shouting at them to go home, and before long, skirmishes broke out and the cops moved in, beating the protesters with their billy clubs. Blood flowed in the streets. Four days after turning twelve years old, I was convinced that the world was breaking apart at the seams.

Do I really have to grow up? I asked my mother as we lay there watching the mayhem.

My mother shrugged. *Beats the alternative,* she said.

I wanted to hide under the covers, make the world go away, but even the comforts of home were beginning to disappear.

Say, you can't go to Michigan Shores from now on, my mother announced casually one day at breakfast. *We don't belong there anymore.*

This was terrible news. I loved that grand old place with its Tudor façade and circular driveway, a social club where we'd belonged since moving back from Connecticut. Patty and I took swim lessons from a man named Gil Finney. They had a bowling alley and a ballroom overlooking Lake Michigan with a huge crystal chandelier. On the rare occasions that we would all go out to eat, it was usually to the dining room of the Michigan Shores Club for special celebrations like First Holy Communions, confirmations, Easter dinners, and at Christmastime. While Holmer and my mother sipped their martinis, we guzzled Shirley Temple cocktails and cherry Cokes until our stomachs gurgled. A man with a paper hat carved huge slabs of rare roast beef that he slipped onto our heated plates with a ladleful of au jus and dollops of creamy horseradish. We feasted on twice-baked potatoes, mushrooms stuffed with spinach, asparagus in hollandaise sauce, mountains of shrimp on beds of chipped ice and lemon wedges, and baskets of warm, yeasty rolls with pats of butter with the club's crest stamped into them. For dessert, we had our choice of apple pie à la mode, pecan bars, coconut macaroons, blueberry tarts, or, my favorite, hot fudge sundaes with chopped walnuts, scoops of whipped cream, and a cherry on top.

I couldn't live without all that.

No one ever told us that we were rich, but it felt like we were, even by Wilmette standards. We got pretty much everything we wanted—horseback riding lessons, summer camp, new bikes every year or two. I never heard Holmer or my mother say, "We can't afford that." A cleaning lady came to our house twice a week, and another woman came every few weeks just to do the ironing. We were one of the first families to get a color TV and a second telephone line installed.

My parents took us on family ski trips for a week each winter in Michigan's Upper Peninsula and out west to Colorado for two weeks in the summer. They escaped for a week or two by themselves to someplace exotic—Puerto Rico, Palm Springs, Miami Beach, or New Orleans, leaving us with a sitter. They always brought us back gifts, dolls, fancy soap from their hotel, or a new outfit. Once, they went to Europe with Jake for a month.

We had no sense of money, where it came from, how to get more, how to manage it, or what to do if it ran out. We simply skimmed the aisles at Betty's of Winnetka, Bonwit Teller, or Saks Fifth Avenue, picking out whatever tickled our fancy, and had the clerk bag it and put it on the house charge. We charged everything, even candy. Mary Claire and I would stop at Lyman-Sargent's Pharmacy on our way home from school nearly every day and charge a box of Andes Creme de Menthe Thins on the house account, wolfing them all down before we'd made it home.

Nowhere was our family's opulence on greater display than inside Holmer's walk-in closet. It was jammed with dozens of Brooks Brothers suits, Italian silk ties that he kept on two racks, stacks of neatly laundered Egyptian cotton shirts, silk knee socks that he held up with garters, and more than a dozen pairs of leather wing tips that he stored on cedar shoe trees so they would retain their shape. He wore felt fedoras with pheasant feathers tucked in the bands of grosgrain ribbon, a Burberry trench coat in the spring and fall, and a finely tailored camel hair coat with braided leather buttons in the winter months. Each night, no matter how much he had to drink, he meticulously hung his clothes up on wooden hangers that he had specially made. *Making up for that sailor suit,* Mary Kay suggested.

Hey, Beau Brummell, ease up on the new clothes, my mother said to him more than once. The cleaning lady started coming just once every two weeks and then not at all. We quit the Chicago Athletic Club, too, where Holmer once entertained customers. For the first time, I began to see that we couldn't just buy everything we wanted on a whim. Old habits are hard to break. Holmer started hiding his new suits under their bed, and I began signing Nancy's name on the charge slips for my new hauls.

From what I could tell by listening outside my parents' bedroom door, Holmer's business was not going well. After he sued his former business partner, he got a job as the national sales manager for the prestigious *Journal of the American Medical Association,* where his name appeared on the masthead. That was great for a while, until he got fired, for what I do not know. Before long, he landed another job, overseeing publications for the American College of Chest Physicians. But he got fired from that job, too, and then he developed a bleeding ulcer.

Was it his erratic behavior? His drinking? Both? Whatever the cause, as Holmer approached his midforties, the trajectory of his career was heading in the wrong direction. He had once been such a high roller that he had his own room at the Waldorf Astoria. His cousins came to him for loans. Now he was the one scrambling to pay bills, sharing an office next to the copy machine. One of his cousins hired him to work at his Michigan Avenue advertising agency, a gesture that we suspected was an act of charity, confirmed after one of his kids loudly and derisively announced to Danny on the St. Francis playground, "Our dad had to give your dad a job."

Now we were quitting the Michigan Shores Club. No more swim

lessons. No more cheeseburgers and fries at the Chatterbox, the little diner inside the club. I tried sneaking in anyway one day after school and ordered a chocolate milkshake.

A charge to number sixty-three, please, I told the waitress, looking around nervously. Brain freeze be damned, I sucked down the ice cream drink as fast as I could before she discovered what a little grifter I was.

THE CROWD CLAPPED AND cheered, but I wept as Mary Kay and her Regina Dominican High School classmates promenaded down the aisle in their white caps and gowns that evening in June 1970. *She's graduating, not dying,* my mother leaned over and whispered to me. It felt like something was being lost forever in that existential moment. Our cozy family life—crazy to many from the outside looking in but comfortable and familiar to me—was about to end. Our oldest sister would be heading off to St. Louis for college in late August. The ten of us would never live together again.

If I had my way, I would have preserved us all in amber at that sweet spot of 1970 with the jazz of our family life thumping throughout the house: moppy-headed high school boys in their shiny Camaros and Corvettes racing up the street to pick up my glamorous older sisters, Mungo Jerry blaring from their car stereos. Or maybe Led Zeppelin or the Doors. They'd come sniffing around in such numbers that Holmer gave them nicknames to tell them apart. One was "the Hugger." Another, "the Kisser."

I would miss Mary Kay scrambling to the dinner table from play practice, reciting her lines. I would miss her friends, who would splay out on Mary Kay's bedroom floor listening to records, begging Patty and me to walk on their backs. When they ran out of cigarettes, they'd dispatch us to ride our bikes to the grocery store to buy them Pop-Tarts and packs of Kools, pretending they were for my mother.

Just as I once urged baby Molly to *stay little,* I wanted all of us frozen in time so that we could remain together, forever. The world scared me, and I was frightened of what might happen to Mary Kay—or any of us—when we ventured out. I know now that this was anxiety and my tears that night were not so much a reflection of foolishness or sentimentality, but fear.

The irony is that life was not as rosy as the narrative I had constructed in my mind. Holmer's drinking and subsequent hangover rants were increasing. Nancy's illness was beginning to rage.

She was getting into more trouble, ditching school, getting drunk, and dabbling in street drugs. She was having such a hard time getting out of bed in the morning that my mother would send me or one of my siblings to throw cold water on her, a chore I was only too happy to execute. After months of Nancy's screaming, scratching, kicking, and door slamming, my parents decided to send her away to boarding school at Woodlands Academy of the Sacred Heart in Lake Forest, Illinois. *Let the nuns deal with her,* my mother said.

When Mary Kay arrived home after her first year of college, she seemed distant, curt, and distracted. She wasn't like her old self, the playful, theatrical big sister who helped us organize backyard carnivals and decorated our playroom like a circus. Mary Kay had a new boyfriend at school and couldn't wait to get back to campus to see him. She announced that she would not be going on our family vacation to Colorado that August. She said she needed to stay home and work to make money for school.

Decades later, I would learn the real reason.

Once she'd left for college, Mary Kay realized how exciting it was to be free from all of us. For the first time in memory, she didn't have to look after her seven younger siblings. She was relieved of her usual oldest sister duties: driving us to play practices or baseball games, picking up the playroom, doing the dishes, or sweeping the kitchen floor. She didn't have to worry about Holmer going ballistic and hitting the nearest kid if he found the house a mess when he came home from work.

Mary Kay finally had freedom to do what she wanted, when she wanted. And she loved it. Still, those early days of school hadn't been easy. Classes were harder than she'd expected, and she had enrolled in one too many. By mid-fall, she was exhausted, lonely, and having trouble concentrating. Her roommate had a serious boyfriend. So, she was alone most of the time, not really fitting in with one crowd or another. She started having dark thoughts.

Sometimes, waves of sadness would come over her with no warning and no obvious cause. They'd settle over her for days, leaving her too confused to focus but too jittery to sleep. My mother suggested that Mary Kay find someone to talk to at the school counseling center, but the woman she spoke to there wasn't much help. She offered only predictable advice: eat healthy food, get plenty of rest.

The worst days were the ones when she could not see a way out. That was an awful, scary feeling. She felt overwhelmed, unable to figure out how to get all her work done. On those days, just being alive seemed to be a chore. One day, she found herself on the roof of her eight-story dorm, where she would go to sunbathe. She swung her feet over the edge of the roof and stared down at the street.

If I jumped, would it even matter?

She wondered if she might be better off dead.

But by spring, Mary Kay was starting to feel better. She found a crowd of like-minded counterculture thinkers who organized war protests and sit-ins. When she wasn't with them, she'd head over to hang out at her boyfriend's fraternity where sex, drugs, and rock 'n' roll flowed freely.

Coming home that summer to the same demands from all of us sent her into a tailspin again. Mary Kay was working as a waitress at the Pancake House when she began feeling nauseous and tired. She hadn't noticed that she had missed her period.

We didn't discuss sex at home, much less birth control. The closest I ever got to a discussion of any kind of sex education was years earlier when I was in fifth grade. My mother pulled me aside after breakfast to warn me that I would be getting a special lesson at school that day. *You know how your sisters get bad stomach cramps once a month? Well, you're going to see a film strip about that in gym class.* Sure enough, the boys were sent out to the playground while Mrs. Wickerscheim, the school nurse, fired up the projector to show us a filmstrip on menstruation.

According to the narrator, we girls each had fallopian tubes coiled inside us that would start releasing eggs soon. If those eggs were left unfertilized (no mention of how the alternative might happen), they would wash right out of our bodies and into a bloody mess in our underwear.

The idea that she might be pregnant terrified Mary Kay. *This can't be happening*, she thought. This was before home pregnancy tests were available, so the only way for her to confirm her suspicions would be through a test administered by a doctor. A friend helped her find one through Planned Parenthood. When the result came back positive, Mary Kay threw up. How would she tell our parents?

She considered going ahead with her pregnancy and putting the baby up for adoption. But she worried that the trauma of turning over her child to someone else would haunt her for the rest of her life. She debated keeping the baby. But the more she thought about that, the more convinced she was that it would not be fair to the baby. From her years of helping with all of us, Mary Kay knew that babies need constant care and steady supervision, neither of which she could provide, emotionally fragile as she was.

"I was in no way ready to take care of another human being," she recalled more than half a century later.

Abortions were illegal in Illinois then. If that's what she wanted to do, she would have to go to New York. She scheduled her visit for early August during the first week of our family's Colorado vacation. With money her boyfriend wired her and an advance on her paycheck, she bought a plane ticket and made an appointment with a Planned Parenthood clinic.

She was met at the airport in New York by a Planned Parenthood volunteer. They took a bus to the clinic. Mary Kay can't remember exactly where that was but, more than fifty years later, she vividly remembers all the details of the procedure. She recalls lying on a cot in a row with other women. She remembers holding back the hair of the woman lying next to her as the woman vomited into a bowl.

After several hours, Mary Kay was free to go. Back home, bleeding and exhausted, Mary Kay walked into our empty house, trudged up the stairs, and collapsed on her bed. We returned from Colorado a few nights later, clueless about what she'd just been through. If Mary Kay was rattled about the abortion, she showed no signs of it to the rest of us. Another family secret had been swallowed whole, undigested.

Later that week, Nancy headed off to college. I was thrilled to see her go.

MARY KAY HAD BEEN my idol, but my relationship with Nancy was a lot more fraught. Nancy was scrappier, edgier, less filtered. We had some good fun growing up. Sometimes, on summer nights, Nancy and I would sit on the front porch, and she would teach me how to blow smoke rings with her Kool cigarettes. We'd make up songs about the neighbors, including one about the kid who left for California, "Frank the Magic Monkey," sung to the tune of "Puff the Magic Dragon." Nancy gave me driving lessons in the parking lot next to the beach on Northwestern University's campus. Though I was not yet thirteen, she would let me take the wheel while she'd stick her head out of the window belting out Billie Holiday tunes.

But the older Nancy got, the meaner she became. By her junior year of high school, she could be downright vicious, especially if she caught me wearing one of her sweaters or a pair of her earrings. She'd scratch my arms and legs or grab a clump of my hair and try to yank it out. Sometimes, she'd spit at me and tell me that I was ugly.

Nancy's friends would stream into the front door, often stoned or tripping on acid, and head straight to the playroom without saying hello. They threw empty beer cans and their greasy boxes of pizza on the floor and left ashtrays filled with butts, some still smoldering. I viewed them all as menaces, but her friend, the ironically named Joy, scared me the most. Joy would scowl as she brushed by me, looking like she might scratch me, too, just for the fun of it.

From what I could tell, my parents were doing all they could to help Nancy through these rocky teenage years. We didn't discuss what was wrong with her or how to help, but I knew Nancy was seeing my mother's psychiatrist. (So much for conflicts of interest.) He had warned my parents that it was not a good idea to let Nancy attend college far from home.

She was too volatile, he said. But Nancy begged them. More than any-thing, she wanted to go to school in Colorado, where many of her friends were going. *What're you gonna do?* my mother said, shrugging. Nancy got good grades. Mary Kay got to go to the school of her choice. My parents worried that Nancy would become even more depressed if she didn't have the chance to go away to school and experience all the fun that college offered. So, they let her go.

What a lot of college kids loved to do most—particularly in Boulder, Colorado, in the early 1970s—were recreational drugs. Lots of them. Mar-ijuana, cocaine, mescaline, LSD, amphetamines. Nancy tried them all.

LATE ONE NIGHT IN April 1973, in Nancy's sophomore year of college, our phone rang and I could hear my mother's muffled voice telling Holmer that there'd been a car accident. My parents' bedroom was down the hall, so it was not easy to make out all the details. Something about Nancy and California and an abortion. The U.S. Supreme Court had decided the *Roe v. Wade* case months earlier, establishing a woman's right to an abortion, but the procedure was not yet easily accessible and certainly not casually considered, especially in our devout Catholic household.

From what I could hear, Nancy evidently had been on her way to Cal-ifornia to get an abortion when her car skidded off the road. She broke her collarbone but was otherwise okay.

Your sister is coming home, is all my mother had to say about it the next morning. I had lots of questions, but was too afraid to ask. I could see that my parents were upset, and I didn't want to make it any worse for them by asking for details.

A few days later, Nancy was back home with us, apparently no longer pregnant, her arm in a sling. She'd dropped out of school just before the end of her sophomore year at the University of Colorado at Boulder and would be living at home for the foreseeable future. I was a sophomore in high school by then, disappointed at the news of Nancy's early return. Life was a lot calmer when she was far away.

I never asked her what had happened or how she was feeling. We never discussed her abortion. I didn't see then that she was sick and hurting. I only saw the pain she caused our parents, and I resented her for that.

Now, she was home with no school, no job, no plan. Clearly, she was miserable. Her bedroom and the one I shared with Patty were attached by a mutual closet. We could hear Nancy sobbing as she lay in her bed day after day. *You okay?* I'd call out to her, slowly becoming aware that she was sick. *Shut the fuck up!* she'd scream back.

Day after day, week after week, Nancy lay in bed, until one day that June. I was standing in the driveway waiting for my mother to take me for a driving lesson when an ambulance came roaring up our street and stopped right in front of the house. The paramedics jumped out, running past me toward our front door. I could hear Mary Kay and my mother screaming inside, pounding on the door. *Open up. Open up. For God's sake, Nancy, open UP!*

Nancy, I would later learn, had locked herself in the bathroom, swallowed a bottle of sleeping pills, and lay in the tub as the water gushed from the tap. Firefighters had to break down the door with a Halligan bar to get in there to fish her out.

I paced around the front lawn, too scared to go inside and look at what was going on upstairs. Nancy had tried to kill herself several times before by swallowing pills, but she always let someone know what she'd done. This time was different. A few minutes later, the front door burst open, and the paramedics hurried out. I could see Nancy's body strapped to a stretcher. Was she moving? They rushed past me so quickly that I couldn't tell if she was dead or alive.

A few seconds later, my mother marched out, her purse slung over her shoulder. She scanned the front lawn. Her eyes had that laser-focused look like a general surveying the battlefield. She crawled into the station wagon and followed the ambulance as it rushed down Greenwood Avenue toward Evanston Hospital. I would later learn that the paramedics checked Nancy's oxygen levels and tried to get her to respond, but she was not regaining consciousness.

As my mother's station wagon faded in the distance, I sat on the lawn and stared at our house. Had our lucky streak finally ended? Each spin of the cylinder in our family game of Russian roulette somehow always came up empty. We managed to survive one dangerous trick after another. Billy at the beach. *Click.* Mary Kay flipped over in the convertible. *Click.* Patty plunged to the bottom of the lake beneath Uncle Johnny. *Click.* Me lying facedown in the icy waters of northern Wisconsin. *Click. Click. Click.* There are only so many empty chambers before the one with the bullet fires.

Those calamities had been unintentional, consequences of carelessness. This was a willful act. If Nancy wanted to die, she would find a way.

I went inside and called Mary Claire. *Meet me in the alley,* I told her, grabbing a pack of my mother's Kent cigarettes. Then I headed out the door, knowing that nothing at home would ever be the same again.

6

While You Were Out: Grandma Died

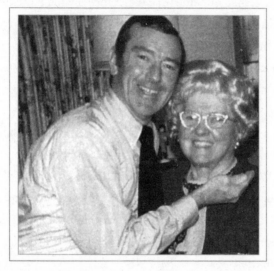

Holmer, the old momma's boy, sitting on
Grandma's lap. Chicago, Illinois, 1973.

Nancy's eyes flickered open as Holmer rubbed her feet.

She looked around the emergency room. *Am I dead?*

No, Holmer said, tears streaming down his cheeks. *No, you are not. Thank God.*

Well, shit, Nancy said and closed her eyes again. Then she started to cry, not because she nearly died but because she didn't.

Once her vital signs were stable, they transferred her upstairs to the psychiatric ward, the same place where my mother had been treated years earlier. Back at home, we resumed our normal pace as if nothing had happened.

Billy and Danny went to summer basketball camp. Molly hopped across the street to play dress-up with the Clohisy sisters. Patty's friends came over to go swimming. Mary Kay and Jake were back at work at the Pancake House. As usual, no one explained why Nancy tried to kill herself this time. Nor did they ask if we had any questions. We were left to try to figure that out on our own. Once again, I was afraid to talk about what had happened, worried that if I asked too many questions, I might upset my parents even more. So, I went back to driver's ed classes, working the cash register at the Kentucky Fried Chicken on Green Bay Road, and drinking beer with my friends at night in the room over Dan Kelly's garage.

But there was an edge to all of us now. Nancy had come *this* close to dying, and we were terrified of what might become of her. Would she try it again? Which one of us would find her dead? I couldn't understand why she would want to die. What does that even feel like? We tried to act normally, but we couldn't just pretend that we didn't see the broken bathroom door where the firefighters rushed in to fish Nancy from the bottom of the tub.

I was fairly certain that everyone on the block had seen the ambulance or heard about it. We could tell by their glances that they knew about Nancy, the way they'd stare at us and then look away when they saw us looking back at them. They probably didn't know what to say.

We were far from being the only family with troubles. A boy in Billy's class drowned in Lake Michigan. The little boy who lived next to our old house died of the flu. A girl in the class between Patty's and mine was killed in a car crash. But no one tried to kill themselves, at least none we knew.

With all eyes on Nancy, Jake was quietly sinking into his own deep depression. He'd been such a gentle, quiet boy that no one expected any trouble out of him.

From the time Jake was a baby, Grandma had pegged him to become a priest. She used to collect pamphlets from various religious orders—Augustinians, Franciscans, Benedictines, Carmelites, and Capuchins—and put them on Jake's dresser, hoping he'd take the bait. Of course, the Jesuits were the gold standard, but Grandma would have settled for Jake becoming a simple diocesan priest. The church relied on its members to propagate the faith. Parents were not only expected to produce a high volume of offspring, they were encouraged to steer one or two of their children toward a religious vocation. A nun here, a priest there. It was the least they could do to thank God for blessing them with so many progeny. Grandma seemed especially motivated, and the way things were going with Mary Kay and Nancy, Jake appeared to be her best shot.

It made sense to me: Father Jake, kindly, thoughtful in his stiff white collar, cradling a baby in his arms at a baptism or carefully sprinkling a coffin with holy water. *May the angels lead you into paradise.* Jake was naturally reverent. Quieter than the rest of us, he kept more to himself, steering clear of our roughhousing and pig piles. He seemed to float above the fray.

Even as a kid, Jake had a strong sense of fairness, speaking up against injustice. He made his way to Washington, D.C., to march in a Vietnam War protest in the spring of his junior year of high school. I could easily see him at the pulpit urging the faithful to be like Christ to others, tend to the poor, comfort the afflicted. *Cause good trouble,* he'd tell them. *Burn your draft cards. Boycott Nestlé.* Real feisty Berrigan brothers stuff.

Holmer and my mother thought Jake should become a doctor, and they encouraged him to declare a premed major. They would have loved to mingle with their friends at cocktail hour and talk about the medical schools that Jake might consider. Success and high achievement were the North Shore way. New Trier East, our public high school, had a reputation for being one of the best in the country. But good Catholics sacrificed and sent their children to Catholic schools, or so we were told. Nearly all graduates of Loyola Academy, the Jesuit high school that Jake attended, also went on to four-year colleges, many to Ivy League schools. Competition was fierce, and expectations were high.

Jake started having trouble sleeping in high school, and, like Nancy and Mary Kay, his anxiety seemed to intensify once he went off to college. Now, as a freshman at John Carroll University, a Jesuit college in suburban Cleveland, Jake was having trouble concentrating in class. Jake was a critical thinker, an Eagle Scout with a sharp eye for details. He could build a fire without using matches, identify animal tracks, and tell you where Saskatchewan was on a map, but he couldn't figure out how to organize his thoughts. Term papers were especially challenging. If he were assigned to write about the Electoral College, for example, he'd know how it was structured and why the votes differ from the popular tally, but he couldn't write it clearly enough for anyone else to understand. After a while, he'd lose sight of what the assignment was, and he'd get too frustrated to write anything.

Students who struggle as Jake did now can get help from individual counselors at the school's writing center. But that service was not available in 1972. It was sink or swim. Jake wasn't just sinking; he was drowning.

It probably didn't help that he was smoking marijuana nearly every day. He started in high school when he and his fellow Pancake House busboys would light up in the alley behind the restaurant. Jake found that pot gave him energy and made him less panicky, but it also clouded his thinking and sapped his motivation.

With his thick black glasses and pocket protectors, Jake looked nothing like your run-of-the-mill stoner. He skewed more nerd—spending hours poring over his almanacs and encyclopedias, memorizing the most arcane facts—motorcycle helmet laws, Incan irrigation systems, the history of the penny.

Now, uncharacteristically, Jake was getting into trouble at school. He and his roommate got expelled from their dorm room for shooting off firecrackers. Jake moved in with a family near campus, staying in a room in their attic. He was horribly lonely there. Jake's insomnia intensified. Sometimes, he felt so drained, it hurt to even blink. Holmer would call Jake and grill him about how school was going. When Jake confessed that he'd skipped a few classes, Holmer would yell into the phone.

Get your goddamn ass out of bed!

Eventually, Jake stopped answering Holmer's calls. My mother suggested that Jake visit the school's counseling center, as she had when Mary Kay began feeling depressed in her freshman year. Jake told the man how lonely he felt and how sluggish he'd become, how he'd toss and turn all night long. He was scared and frustrated as he began to fail one class after another. The counselor's solution? *Join a fraternity. Get drunk. Have more fun.*

Jake didn't know how to have fun, and nothing he was trying was working. After Nancy's suicide attempt that summer, he'd become even more confused and depressed. He was often unable to get more than an hour or two of sleep a night. He'd stumble around during the day in a kind of stupor. But we were all so freaked out about Nancy, few of us took the time to even notice.

Jake went back to campus the next fall more depressed than ever.

I'D NEVER BEEN INSIDE a psych ward before. The attendant pressed the buzzer, and the doors clicked like a pop gun, making me jump. My mother and I walked down the hall and found Nancy sitting in the dayroom, a large area furnished with a few cheap vinyl couches and several plastic chairs scattered around. It had been several days since Nancy locked herself into the bathroom and tried to drown. People shuffled by without looking at one another. A TV mounted on the wall was tuned in to a soap opera, though no one was really watching.

If she saw me coming, she didn't let on. No wave or wink. She just stared straight ahead. I thought Nancy would be in a hospital gown, but she was wearing a pair of blue jeans and an oversize blue-and-white tattersall plaid shirt that I'd been admiring in her closet for some time. She looked a lot smaller here than she did at home. Her face was rounder than I remembered it, and her skin was pasty white against her long, thick, chestnut brown hair. She seemed pretty punchy on whatever drugs they had given her that day, and she didn't even bother to look up at me. All these years later, I can't remember where my mother was during this visit—talking to the doctor or a nurse, maybe.

Hey, I said to Nancy.

No answer.

Nancy reached for her cigarettes and lit one up. The floors were shiny, but the place smelled rancid, a sickening potpourri of vomit, feces, and Pine-Sol.

I didn't know what to say, so I tried making small talk. *How's the food?* She didn't answer. *What's her story?* I said, nodding toward a woman who was rocking back and forth in the corner. Silence. The old Nancy would have already come up with a nickname for that woman, "Whistler's Mother," maybe, something clever and not altogether kind. But this Nancy just stared, no emotion. I noticed the paper slippers on Nancy's feet and tried making a little joke.

Can you get those things monogrammed?

She turned her back to me.

Nancy and I just sat there. I wish now that I would have taken that opportunity to ask her how she was feeling, to let her know that I was glad she was still alive. Did she want to tell me about why she tried to kill herself? God knows, I was curious enough. *Did she really want to die?* It might have been a big relief for her to talk about it. And then I would have understood better, too. Maybe I wouldn't have been so angry at her.

There was so much more I could have said, like, *What can I do to help you feel better?* Maybe then she wouldn't have felt as lonely or out of options. She would have seen how much I loved her.

But I didn't say any of that. I was fifteen years old, and I was still angry with her for trying to kill herself at the same time that my mother promised to give me a driving lesson. And now she was giving me the cold shoulder after I took the time on a summer day to come and see her in the hospital.

So, I started watching the soap opera from the TV on the ceiling. *All My Children.* So much easier to get taken in by the drama on the screen than the one playing out at home. After several more minutes, my mother returned, and we left. Nancy and I didn't bother to say goodbye to each other.

Not long after that, Nancy came home. Our parents still offered no explanation about what had happened or advice about how we should act toward her, what we should say and do or—more important—what we should not say or do. We still didn't know why she did this. I was terrified that she would do it again.

At first, Nancy mostly stayed in her bedroom, even at dinnertime. The medication made her too groggy to stand for long or carry on much of a conversation. When she did come downstairs, she was often rude and selfish, leaving a mess in the kitchen, making hurtful remarks. By mid-September, it was clear that she was not going back to college.

Nancy embarrassed us. No one I knew had a sister who was sick like this, lying in bed most of the day with some strange illness that had no name, couldn't be seen on an x-ray or confirmed through blood tests. One doctor said Nancy had schizophrenia. Another said it was mania with depression. Holmer wondered if her wild mood swings were caused by all the street drugs she took at college. *They scrambled her brain,* he said.

Whatever it was, she wasn't getting better, and the doctors said she might never recover. The uncertainty had us all on edge. The mood at home grew so tense that it felt at times like our house had been doused in gasoline and could blow up any second. We started to turn on each other, fighting over the slightest things—which show to watch on TV, who got to sit where on the couch. *Don't hog the phone. Who left the empty milk bottle in the refrigerator?* We couldn't relax. I had a hard time concentrating on my homework.

After months of Nancy shuffling around the house, picking fights, sobbing in her bed, raiding the liquor cabinet, and overdosing on more pills, my parents decided that she needed long-term care, regardless of the cost.

She left for the Menninger Clinic in November 1974, my senior year of high school. I was relieved to have her out of the house. The facility was founded in Topeka, Kansas, in 1925 by Sigmund Freud disciples Karl Menninger and his brother, William. This world-famous psychiatric hospital was featured in magazines as one of the nation's premier mental institutions, catering to captains of industries, World War II veterans suffering from post-traumatic stress, and movie stars like Gene Tierney. *It's quite an exclusive program,* my mother said, as if Nancy had been accepted at Smith or Vassar.

Just as her mother took comfort in knowing that Uncle Johnny was being well cared for when he was sent away to St. Coletta in 1949, my mother was consoled by the notion that Nancy would be getting some of the best care in the world. She wasn't dispatching Nancy like a biting dog to the pound.

In my naivete, I imagined those doctors would fix Nancy in no time. She would come back sassier, funnier, and cleverer than ever.

Insurance covered none of it, of course. Though, clearly, Nancy was in danger of dying, mental illnesses were not considered to be as worthy of treatment like other diseases. If you needed psychiatric care, you had two choices: pay for it yourself or go to a state institution. I knew that the Menninger Clinic was expensive and that my parents didn't have the kind of money anymore to pay for that and for our schooling at Regina Dominican, the Catholic all-girls school where Patty and I were enrolled. The two of us decided to pay our tuition with money we made working nights and weekends as waitresses at the local Howard Johnson's restaurant. Four hundred bucks each was a lot of money then. I was secretly hoping the gesture alone would be enough to impress my parents, and we wouldn't really have to follow through on it. But they lunged at the offer. My sacrifice only made me resent Nancy more.

The Menninger brothers were famous for identifying many of the illnesses now outlined in the *Diagnostic Statistical Manual,* the so-called bible of psychiatric disorders, but the doctors there came up empty on how to treat my sister or even what her diagnosis was. Nancy escaped a few times in her first months by simply walking out the door.

She eloped, I heard my mother tell Holmer the first time the hospital called, and for a few minutes, I thought Nancy had gotten married. I didn't know that's what they called it when a patient walks away against doctor's orders. Each time, the Topeka police found her and sent her back. But she wasn't getting better. Her fancy treatment didn't work after all.

Four months and tens of thousands of dollars later, Nancy came home for good, saying she couldn't stand living in the institution. *They're all nuts,* she said with a straight face. Nancy enrolled in a day program at a hospital on Chicago's north side. Against all ethical standards, she started dating one of the doctors there, a resident named Henry, whom we thought looked like John Sebastian from the Lovin' Spoonful. He came on one of our family ski trips. We all wished that she would marry him someday and live happily ever after.

MIDWAY THROUGH MY SENIOR year of high school, my own world started to crumble, right on cue. First Mary Kay, then Nancy, then Jake. Now, it was my turn. Nancy's return from the Menninger Clinic was making me nervous. She was meaner and more physically abusive than ever, throwing shoes at my head, jabbing my ribs with her elbow, spitting at me, scratching my arms and legs. She chased me around the breakfast room table with a steak knife one afternoon, and I escaped by running upstairs and locking myself in the bathroom. A few days later, I woke up to find her standing over my bed with a carving knife in her hand. When I looked at her, I didn't see someone who was suffering. I saw someone who could kill me. She scared the hell out of me.

I was desperate to get out of that house.

I'd been excited about going off to college and had set my sights on Northwestern University, where I would study journalism. The summer before, I'd been accepted to Northwestern's exclusive high school journalism institute and given a scholarship. So, I figured I'd be a shoo-in. I always loved writing. Even as I struggled with math and science, I could count on my English classes to give me a platform to express myself.

The mid-1970s were heady days for journalists. The Watergate hearings were just wrapping up, and soon Richard Nixon would resign—all because of an investigation begun by two enterprising young *Washington Post* reporters. I was going to follow in their footsteps and light the world on fire with my reporting, too.

The letter from Northwestern's admissions office arrived on a Friday afternoon, and, judging from how thin the envelope was, I knew before I ripped it open that I had been rejected. My shoulders started to shake as I scanned the page and the words began to sink in: "We regret that we are not able to offer you admission." *This can't be,* I thought. *I have to go there. I need to go there.* My friends were getting into their dream schools. *Do these jerks in admissions not know how hard I work?*

I marched upstairs and put on my mother's best Diane von Fursten-berg dress, a string of pearls, and a pair of espadrilles and, with Patty at the wheel, took off in the family station wagon for the admissions office. *This isn't a good idea,* Patty said. But I had never been shy about taking matters into my own hands.

The year before, when the orthodontist had yet to remove my braces, despite several promises to do so and junior prom fast approaching, I took some wire cutters and a pair of pliers and did the job myself. The orthodontist stared at my mouth in disbelief on my next visit. In forty years of practice, he'd never seen a kid take off her own braces. *Get in here,* he called to his assistant. Then the two of them put a new set of braces right back on and adjusted the bill accordingly. If I could take off my own braces, I could sweet-talk my way into Northwestern.

Sorry, the admissions officer said. *This is a world-class school, highly competitive, and your grades and test scores just aren't good enough.* Not good enough. I stood up to leave, those words ringing in my ears.

Patty was waiting for me in the parking lot when I stormed out. I jumped in the car and slammed the door so hard we both thought it might fall off.

Now what?

I had to get out of that house. At the same time, I was terrified of what might become of me if I left home. Look what had happened to each of my older siblings when they came back from college. Mary Kay grew distant. Nancy and Jake dropped out and were now so confused and depressed that they could barely get out of bed. Would that happen to me, too?

I didn't have anyone to talk to about my fears. I had alienated most of my friends by being so irritable and angry. Mary Kay had moved out of the house into an apartment in the city after she graduated. My parents certainly weren't any help. As far as I was concerned, they were a major part of the problem. Even Patty seemed to be of little use to me anymore. Our Tiger Pit adventures were long over, and the space between our beds was more of a gulf. We barely spoke. I resented her and her straight A report cards, how everything seemed to come so easily to her. In a rage one day, I grabbed clumps of Patty's clothes and threw them out the window. It didn't make any sense to turn on Patty, the one person who always stood up for me and tried to make me feel better about myself. She hadn't done anything wrong. But nothing made sense to me any longer. Hurt people hurt people, as the saying goes. Just as Nancy treated me cruelly, I started doing the same to Patty.

I was so surly that even I hated me. My mother was at a loss.

What's gotten into you? she asked one afternoon as I pushed Patty out of the way on my way to the kitchen sink. *Are you pregnant?*

Pregnant! Just the idea of that made me feel like my head would explode. I couldn't breathe. I couldn't see. The truth is, I could have been. I would never admit to that, of course. Good girls don't have sex. At least that's what the nuns told us. And I was a very good girl.

I was working hard to pay my own tuition, going to Mass each Sunday and even some days during the week. I was a class officer, Piglet in our school's production of *Winnie the Pooh,* the features editor of our student newspaper. I even joined the math club, though, admittedly, that was only because Mary Claire and I had a contest to see how many pictures each of us could get into the yearbook. Sure, I smoked cigarettes and drank beer. (Lots of beer.) But I didn't smoke pot or do other drugs. Drugs scared me. I was not going to crack up the way I'd seen my siblings do after they started taking street drugs.

Even if I could have figured out a way to access birth control, I would never have done so. That would be admitting that my boyfriend and I were having sex. I wasn't about to do that, not to a doctor, not to my mother, not to my best friends, not even—bizarrely—to myself.

Growing up with so many unexplained and unexplored traumas—an emotionally distant mother who leaves mysteriously, a physically abusive father who drinks too much, a knife-wielding sister—I'd learned how to block out what I didn't want to think or hear or see. When you put on blinders, it becomes easy to create your own reality, to blur fact with fiction. You sharpen the focus to only a few pixels so that you can't see the whole picture. You start to wonder if something really happened or if you were making it up. After a while, I couldn't trust myself to know the difference.

Oh my God, I thought as my mother and my youngest sister, Molly, now ten years old, stared at me. *Am I pregnant?* My period, which was always regular, heavy, and excruciatingly painful, was now two days late. I'd been checking my underwear every few minutes, hoping for the slightest drop of blood. *Holy shit,* I thought. *Now what? What am I going to do?*

I could throw myself down the basement stairs. A coat hanger? I had no idea the precise mechanics of how to do such a thing. *Oh my God! Could this really be happening?*

Even as I was terrified of this possibility, I was livid at my mother for accusing me of such a thing. How dare she! The fact that she thought that I might be pregnant must mean that she considered me to be no better than Nancy. If I was like Nancy, then I must be crazy, too. What was to stop me from ending up in a mental hospital, wearing paper slippers, lying in bed all day, getting fat on medication that made my mouth dry and eyes glassy?

The next thing I knew, I was swinging my arms wildly, punching the walls, throwing a chair, kicking and screaming. I felt like I was in a kind of fugue state, watching myself from the ceiling, unable to stop. All the fear and rage and confusion were flying out of my body.

My mother ran to the phone and did the only thing she knew to gain control of a situation like this. She called the cops.

Two officers arrived a few minutes later and came into the kitchen to ask me some questions. By then, I'd collapsed, exhausted, lying on the floor, sobbing. Had I taken any drugs? *No.* Did I feel like hurting myself? *No.* Did I feel like hurting my mother? My brothers? My little sister over there? *No, I said. No. I'm sorry. I'm so sorry.* Now my mother was crying, something I don't ever remember seeing her do, not when Nancy was carted off in that stretcher, not during the worst of Holmer's tirades, not ever.

Was I turning into Nancy with these wild mood swings? How many times had I seen her fly into fits of rage like this? Now, I was just as fierce. Had I lost my mind, too?

After a few minutes, the cops left, and that was the end of that. No more questions, no explanations or suggestions that I should talk to a doctor or see a therapist. My shift at the restaurant was starting soon. So, I headed out the back door and walked the eight blocks to work, relaxing a bit with each step. Twenty minutes later, blinders back on, I was scurrying around the restaurant, smiling at customers, taking their orders, delivering milkshakes and clam rolls, doing my best to hide the ugly truth of what had just happened at home.

The next day, I woke up to menstrual cramps so intense that I thought I was being stabbed. That blinding pain had never felt so welcome.

My mother took me to the gynecologist a few weeks later so I could get on birth control pills. I'd been diagnosed with endometriosis. Being on the Pill would lessen the intensity of my menstrual cramps and help regulate my moods. But my mother and I knew the other reason why it was good for me to be on the Pill, even if neither of us would actually say it.

Shortly after that, my mother told me she thought I should apply to DePauw University in Greencastle, Indiana, a little town fifty miles west of Indianapolis. Some of her friends' kids went there and loved it. I had never heard of the place. Besides, it was late March, and I had already been accepted at the University of Missouri, an excellent school for journalism.

No, my mother said. *You'll be better off as a big fish in a little pond.* So, I applied and got in. They gave me a scholarship, even though I spelled the name of the school wrong on my application. Not a big scholarship but a scholarship nonetheless. I had to read the letter twice. I was good enough for them.

I ARRIVED IN GREENCASTLE a little after noon on August 23, 1975, the day after my eighteenth birthday, with the worst hangover of my life.

What had sounded so noble the night before—eighteen beers, one for each year—now, in the clear light of a blazing sun, seemed just plain stupid. The campus was pretty enough with its redbrick Georgian buildings, the imposing and iconic East College tower, and lush green lawns. But the town left a lot to be desired for my North Shore Chicago sensibilities. Corn silos everywhere but not a suitable boutique to be found. What passed for the area's fine dining featured garlic cheeseburgers, oversize sodas served in huge red plastic glasses, and pork tenderloin sandwiches "as big as your head."

Not the place for me, I told my parents, still feeling quite queasy. *Let's turn around and go home now.* But it was too late. They were madly unpacking my stuff in hopes of getting on the road for the four-hour trip back to Chicago.

I resigned myself to making do there for the time being. Later that day, stumbling around campus for the first time, I saw a sign reading FREE BEER taped to a tree. Instinctually, I followed the arrow, eager for a little hair on the tail of the dog that had bit me the night before. It turned out to be a false claim by the students who ran the college newspaper. DePauw, founded by Methodists, was officially a dry campus, I learned to my horror. I signed up to join the newspaper staff anyway and got my first assignment that same day, a roundup of the incoming freshmen's impressions of campus. For the better part of the next four years, I spent most of my time in that building, smoking cigarettes, eating garlic cheeseburgers, gossiping about interoffice romances, and sleeping off hangovers on the broken-down couch in the corner of the newsroom that we affectionately named "the Green Whore."

College life was providing me with the escape I craved, the acceptance I searched for, and the structure I desperately needed.

NANCY, ON THE OTHER hand, was going from bad to worse.

She tried to kill herself again that fall and again just before Christmas 1975 by swallowing yet another bottle of sleeping pills. (Why weren't my parents locking up these damn pills?) We all got through the holidays, and on the day after New Year's, they drove her to Chicago-Read Mental Health Center, the state-run hospital, formerly known as Dunning and, before that, the County Insane Asylum and Infirmary.

Medical records I obtained years later from an open records request describe Nancy as a "white, single, very attractive 22-year-old woman who appears much younger than her age." They note that Nancy had recently tried to kill herself by swallowing pills, and my parents were worried that she might try to kill herself again.

I imagine Holmer and my mother were greatly troubled to have to take Nancy to this facility, but they had no choice. She had just spent several weeks for yet another stint at Evanston Hospital's psych ward, and they had no money left for private care. The notes show that Nancy had a hard time at Read. The attending nurse reported that one night a little more than a week into her eighteen-day stay, Nancy was "crying and squealing," afraid that her body "was breaking apart."

The next day, one of the social workers wrote:

Nancy appears to be a very immature young woman with little insight into her problems, i.e. things just happen to her and she is unable to see her role in creating her own situations. She is a very dependent, needy person who seemingly manipulates others by playing a very helpless role.

Well, yes, she was needy, you idiot, I thought when I read those notes years later. *She had serious mental illness. That's why she was in a damn hospital.* The medical staff noted that Nancy was hearing voices, had a distorted body image and very low self-esteem, and was preoccupied with thoughts of suicide. They wondered if she was suffering from hysterical psychosis, an emotional reaction to a traumatic event. The notes do not specify what that traumatic event may have been. She reported "multiple drug problems," but the chart didn't list any specifics.

Under medical history, the staff referenced her many suicide attempts and that she had been at the Menninger Clinic for four months the previous year. They also noted that Nancy had come home just before the end of her sophomore year at the University of Colorado but made no mention of her car accident or the abortion.

It was clear from the notes that the staff considered Nancy a pest. The night after squealing and crying, Nancy went to the nurses' station "demanding aspirin." When she was told she could not have any because there were no orders from the doctor for that, Nancy "became agitated." The nurse injected her with fifty milligrams of chlorpromazine, an antipsychotic. "The patient was put in the Quiet Room to rest," the note said.

They diagnosed Nancy as having a "typical case of depressive neurosis/ schizophrenia/schizo-effective [sic] disorder." In other words, the kitchen sink. In other words, blah blah blah, gobbledygook that went no further in helping anyone understand her, then or now.

They said her prognosis was "rather poor."

A FEW WEEKS AFTER Nancy was discharged from Read, I returned to my dorm after class to find a pink slip with the words WHILE YOU WERE OUT tucked into my mail slot. The woman who answered the phone lines handed it to me with a wince. *Uh-oh,* I thought. *Now what?* Apparently, my mother had called while I was gone. She left only a two-word message: *Grandma died.*

My eyes filled with tears. Grandma? She died? I dashed down the hall to the phone booth and had the operator return the call.

Mom, really? You left that message with the operator?

Yeah, well, my mother said. *Sorry about that. It's been busy around here, and I had SO many people to call.*

I wasn't expecting her to send a grief counselor. Grandma was eighty-four years old, living in a nursing home since Grandpa died four years earlier. Always eccentric, Grandma had been getting even battier, staying in bed most of the day, asking odd questions like what day my mother washed corsets and if someone would please bring her some of that "nice Jesuit wine." (It was ten o'clock in the morning!)

Still, I thought my mother could have delivered the news with a little more sensitivity. She never spoke ill of Grandma to us, even though Grandma repeatedly called her Joan, the name of Holmer's old girlfriend, but we could read my mother's body language. We had a framed picture of Grandma that we took out and displayed atop our living room secretary each time she would come to visit. The minute that old lady left our house to go back to Milwaukee, my mother would snap the frame shut and shove the picture back into the drawer, where it would remain until Grandma's return.

Now, she would never return. Apparently, while I was out, Grandma died. Something about the way that message was worded suggested a causal relationship that made me feel guilty, like, if I hadn't so callously gone off to my Intro to Poli Sci class, Grandma would still be with us. Of course, I wasn't to blame. I knew that. But our family's shorthand way of dealing with these situations—by simply not discussing them or making light of it—had an insidious way of fueling shame and blame where none was warranted.

I STUDIED ABROAD DURING the first semester of my junior year, eager for the chance to get even farther away from home and see the world. The course was geared to political science and economics majors to compare and contrast Western countries and those behind the Iron Curtain. I imagined that living in Vienna and Budapest would be thrilling. Who wouldn't love traveling by train on weekends and holidays to see the castles and palaces of Austria, Oktoberfest in Munich, gondola rides in Venice, the Sistine Chapel? But the more breathtaking the sights, the more intensely homesick I became. I thought the adventures of traveling through Europe would give me a welcome distance from all the commotion of my family. Instead, they made me miss them all that much more. I worried about how everyone was holding up. What if something terrible happened while I was thousands of miles away? It may seem counterin-tuitive, but, I've come to learn, people who live through trauma like the kind our family experienced tend to develop anxiety about being away. We become deeply vigilant.

I know what I'll do, I thought one sparkling autumn day as I hiked the Alps near Innsbruck. *I'll move up my flight home and surprise them all for Christmas.* It'll be just like that Lennon Family Christmas special they show every year on PBS. The whole family weeps with joy when the son comes marching onstage decked out in his Vietnam War uniform to sur-prise his mother. Only, this time, I'll be the star of the show.

Mary Kay can pick me up at O'Hare airport, and I'll walk in the front door on Christmas Eve, just about the time that my mother will be head-ing downstairs with her tower of wrapped presents. The family room fire-place will be crackling, and the living room fireplace will be aglow. Bing Crosby, or maybe Frank Sinatra, will be crooning on the stereo. Danny and Billy and Molly will be playing a spirited game of table hockey while Jake and Patty and Nancy sip eggnog and chat by the fire. Then we'll all line up for a picture, the way we always do on Christmas Eve, and wait for the timer on Holmer's camera to click.

Shit! he'll yelp as the camera snaps precisely at the wrong time, captur-ing an image of his backside and not the ten of us huddled by the tree.

We'll all howl with delight.

Then we'll break out Holmer's holiday punch and spike it with rum. No rum for Holmer, though. Not anymore. He quit drinking a few months earlier after he was arrested for drunk driving in New Jersey on one of his business trips. We were never told the details, of course.

We only knew that there was trouble and Holmer would not be home for a few more days. Many years later, Holmer let us all know that the night he spent in jail was enough to convince him that, as much as he loved the taste of booze and the way it made him feel, he just couldn't drink it any-more. It was killing him. How many jobs had he lost because of his erratic behavior? Now, all the alcohol was burning a hole in his gut.

He joined Alcoholics Anonymous, or, as Holmer jokingly referred to it, "the Lodge." When the urge to drink came upon him, Holmer called his sponsor, sometimes four or five times a day. Now, on his business trips to New York, instead of heading to nightclubs in Harlem, he searched for an AA meeting, most often at St. Patrick's Cathedral on Fifth Avenue.

Well, there goes all my fun, my mother sighed when Holmer declared that he'd had his last drop of drink. Their marriage had been bathed in booze for a quarter of a century. Alcohol had soothed their nerves through colicky newborns and dying parents and business deals that suddenly fell apart. It settled them down as they ventured from Milwaukee to Chicago to Connecticut and back to Chicago, gaining a kid or two with each move. When the going got tough, they headed to the liquor cabinet, and, suddenly, they weren't so weak or afraid anymore.

Liquid courage: Stingers and martinis. White Russians and Rob Roys. Grasshoppers and gimlets. Gin and tonic and Beefeaters. Mimosas and Bloody Marys. Johnnie Walker, neat. Crème de menthe. Each drink more delicious than the last.

Holmer was famous for his drunken antics. Once while he was in New Orleans for a medical convention, he jumped up onstage at a stripper bar. *It's okay,* he announced. *I'm a gynecologist.* And there was the time Mary Kay looked out of the window of her college dorm room during St. Louis University's parents weekend and saw Holmer streaking naked across the lawn. After a night of carousing, Holmer frequently drove his Cutlass convertible on people's lawns to drop them off, announcing, *Door-to-door service!* as my mother sat giggling beside him.

Each week, Schaefer's Liquor Store would deliver bottles of gin and vermouth and a quarter keg of Hamm's beer that Holmer kept on tap in our basement refrigerator. He taught Uncle Johnny and the rest of us how to pour the perfect headless beer and serve it to him with a salute.

Now what? my mother wondered. All their friends loved to drink just as much as they did. Would this kill their social life? My parents belonged to a dinner club that met once a month—eight couples who took turns hosting bacchanalian feasts that stretched long into the night. When it was my parents' turn to host, Patty and I would sit on the top of the stairs and listen to them telling saucy stories, their boozy voices rolling up the stairs. We once woke up on a Sunday morning to find one of the men, the father of nine, sprawled facedown on the living room floor, a pitcher of whiskey sours at his side.

Holmer now went to AA meetings almost every day. He pored over his Friend of Bill W. books, underlining whole sections on how to turn your life over to a higher power, surrender to the will of one greater than you.

"I was fertile ground for alcoholism," Holmer scribbled on a piece of paper he tucked into the book's pages. "Alcohol was the key thing in my life. I depended on it."

Holmer encouraged us all to go to Al-Anon meetings for the families of alcoholics and learn the mantras that he was saying to get his life straightened up.

Easy does it.

First things first.

Keep coming back.

It works if you work it.

Keep it simple, stupid.

I went to a few meetings and found it inspiring to see that Holmer was trying so hard to break the choke hold that alcohol had on him, one that had already derailed his once promising career. And I was proud of him for wanting to take control of his life. He seemed energized by the challenge. But I had no plans to give up my own precious beer.

Nancy seemed headed in the right direction, too. She sent me a letter a few weeks after I arrived in Vienna letting me know that she got a job as an assistant to a music teacher at a public school in Chicago. She found a little apartment in Chicago's Lakeview neighborhood and had a serious boyfriend whom she was hoping to marry.

"Write back soon and tell me all there is to tell about your adventures," she wrote. "P.S. Can we correspond?"

I was stunned by her cheerful note. How could this be? Medication? Therapy? Both? Had Nancy finally found a way to break the grip of her dark thoughts and wild behavior? She sounded so chipper, just like the Nancy from the old days. *Can we correspond?* Classic Nancy, tongue in cheek. I was excited to see her again at Christmas.

My plane arrived on time, and I got through customs without breaking any of the little wooden Christmas ornaments that I bought for my mother. The second I saw Mary Kay standing at her car waiting for me, I knew something terrible had happened. She could barely look me in the eyes.

It's bad, she said as I slid into the passenger's seat. Nancy had cut off her hair a few days earlier and tried to kill herself again by swallowing another bottle of pills. Mary Kay had to drag Nancy down the block by her armpits to get her to the emergency room. Now Nancy was back in the psych ward on suicide watch. *No way will she be home for Christmas,* Mary Kay said.

As I look back on this now, I see that a more sensitive person would be alarmed, worried sick about this poor woman who keeps trying to kill herself. *Poor Nancy! What can I do to help my sister?* I might have thought. But no. Instead, I was angry. Nancy had screwed up my dramatic homecoming plans. Once again, she was stealing all the oxygen in the room.

This was not the Currier and Ives scene I had spent weeks imagining. Of course it wasn't. How could I have been so stupid to think it would be anything but chaos with this family? Nancy would always find a way to make a mess of things. Four months away wasn't going to magically alter that reality.

Holmer was steam cleaning the living room carpet when I walked in the door. My mother was upstairs, sipping her martini as she wrapped her last-minute presents.

Hey, whatta you know? Look who's home early, my mother slurred.

The rest of the family was scattered, in their rooms, sulking.

I had been right about one thing: Bing Crosby warbled through our living room stereo. *Oh by gosh, by golly. It's time for mistletoe and holly.*

. . .

A FEW WEEKS LATER, Nancy moved home yet again, and by the next summer, she was back to her old ways, barely getting out of bed. It had been
five years since she'd come home from Colorado and tried to drown herself in the girls' bathroom. Despite hundreds of hours of therapy and
months in various hospitals, she only seemed to be getting worse.

We lost count how many times she tried to kill herself by swallowing
pills. The antipsychotic drugs she was taking now, Haldol and Stelazine,
made her joints stiff and her mouth dry. Her brown eyes, once so clear,
were cloudy. She was dizzy, nauseated, and had trouble peeing. She sometimes rambled nonsense or lay in bed howling. She seemed more like a
zombie than the girl she had been just a few years earlier—a sassy boy-
crazy teenager in Villager shirtdresses and Capezio flats who told her
friends that all she really wanted to do was to find a cute guy, settle down,
and raise a family.

That summer, I was working as a secretary at a small marketing firm
on Chicago's Gold Coast that Mary Kay and her business partner ran.
Many nights, I stayed at Mary Kay's apartment near Lincoln Park. After
work, we'd spend evenings listening to albums, waxing our arms, making
taco salads. This was just before my senior year of college. After keeping
us all at a distance for some years, Mary Kay seemed to be warming up
to the family again. I loved getting fashion tips from her, hearing stories
about her romances.

When I called home one morning in June and Nancy answered, I
could tell right away that she was in a foul mood.

Mom there?

Nope, Nancy said, sounding groggy.

Where is she?

How the hell do I know?

Do you know when she'll be back?

Nope.

Mary Kay's twenty-sixth birthday was coming up, and she was throwing a party at her new apartment. I was calling to let my mother know

that I was planning on staying at Mary Kay's that night and probably for the rest of the weekend, too.

What's the matter with you? I asked Nancy.

Fuck you, Nancy said and hung up. Those were the last words my sister ever spoke to me.

7

We All Have to Go Sometime

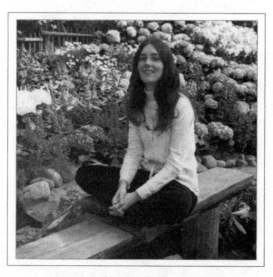

Nancy, Highland Park, Illinois, 1972.

Friday, June 16, 1978, was hot and sticky in Chicago, with the threat of thunderstorms looming.

Nancy had been so sweet that morning, helping Billy with the fingering for his guitar chords. She knew the therapeutic value of music and how it could help him ride out the strange waves of sadness that had begun to wash over him earlier that spring. Just as all of us had struggled in those later high school years, Billy, now seventeen, was feeling a bit lost and confused. He had no obvious reason to be unhappy. That's what made this so unsettling.

Billy had plenty of friends, and he was handsome enough to attract lots of romantic interest. Despite my parents' earlier worries that he would turn out to be a troublemaker, Billy was blossoming into more of the kind of kid every parent would want. His grades were excellent. He made the varsity basketball team and had just been elected vice president of his senior class at New Trier East High School. Holmer nicknamed him "the Happy Jock." Colleges from across the country were sending him mail urging him to apply.

Despite this, Billy, like the rest of us, sometimes doubted himself, wondering if he was good enough. A left-hander, he was fumbling with some minor chords at the breakfast table when Nancy came downstairs from her bedroom that morning. *Try it like this,* Nancy said, moving one of Billy's fingers higher up on the guitar's neck. Her advice worked. Now, Billy's chord sounded crisper. He wished he could stay and jam with Nancy a bit longer, but he needed to get to work stocking shelves at the grocery store.

A little after noon, Billy hopped on his bike and headed off.

Nancy was twenty-four years old now. Her friend Joy and the rest of her crew of wild high school friends were long gone. Most had graduated from college and were settling down. They rented apartments in the fashionable sections of Lakeview and Lincoln Park that they decorated with Pier 1 pillows and dishes from Crate & Barrel. On Saturday nights, they got drunk on margaritas or strawberry daiquiris at Butch McGuire's on Division Street and met for Sunday brunch at trendy restaurants with funny names like Great Gritzbe's Flying Food Show or Lawrence of Oregano. Some of her friends were engaged to be married, others were married already, having babies. They were living the life that Nancy wanted, but she knew, with each passing day, she likely would never have.

Word had gotten around that Nancy "kinda lost it," an old boyfriend of hers—the one we called "the Kisser"—told me years later. He ran into her in front of her apartment sometime in the late spring of 1976, but barely recognized her. Nancy invited him in to see her place, which was a bit of a wreck, piles everywhere.

"I could tell she wasn't right," he said. Nancy, once so cute and cheerful, looked bloated and foggy.

Let's get together again, Nancy said to him.

But they never did.

She moved home a few weeks later.

Hour after hour, she lay in bed staring at her bedroom ceiling, weighed down by medication that may have controlled her wild outbursts and helped her to sleep but did nothing to cure her.

Only Ellen, her science fair buddy, came to visit now. Nancy once showed Ellen the diary she kept, spelling out all the reasons why she wanted to die.

You don't mean that, Nancy, Ellen said.

Yes, I do, Nancy said.

Earlier that week, Holmer found Nancy sobbing in her room. She told him she was tired of trying to kill herself with pills. It wasn't working. She just wanted to get the job done, to be out of her misery once and for all. *If I can find the nerve to do it, I'm just going to jump in front of a train,* Nancy said.

The very idea that Nancy would consider such a desperate and violent act rattled Holmer so much that he started to weep. *Oh, Nanny, please,* he said, calling her by her nickname. *Things will get better, I promise. Let's take it one day at a time.*

Early in the afternoon of Billy's impromptu guitar lesson, Nancy reached for tranquilizers and stuffed as many pills as she could into her mouth. My mother found her passed out in her bed and the empty bottle on her bedroom floor. She called 911. The paramedics, by now familiar with Nancy's routine, rushed over and pumped her stomach. They gave her charcoal pills to absorb any excess toxins. The dose she'd taken was not enough to kill her, they told my mother.

If you want us to take her to the emergency room, we'll need to charge you, one of the paramedics said. My mother knew from experience that an ambulance ride might cost them hundreds, potentially thousands, of dollars. She and Holmer were still paying off hefty bills for Nancy from the Menninger Clinic and various Chicago hospitals. Just a few months earlier, they had to pay a private duty nurse to be on suicide watch, monitoring Nancy around the clock; when that got too expensive, they took turns doing it themselves.

They never sat down and tallied the cost of the dozen or more hospital stays for Nancy and her psychiatry bills over the past ten years, but it had wiped out their savings. Now, another bill? *No thanks,* my mother told the paramedics that afternoon. *We'll take it from here.* Then, she signed a release, acknowledging that she was assuming full responsibility for Nancy's safety and well-being.

Patty, who was going into her sophomore year of nursing school at Marquette University, was home that day, waiting for her afternoon waitressing shift to begin. She helped my mother take care of Nancy after the paramedics left. Patty made Nancy a ham-and-cheese sandwich, hoping it would settle her stomach. When Nancy threw that up, Patty, true to her nickname, Yygor, dutifully cleaned up the mess. She stayed at Nancy's side for most of the afternoon, making small talk, reading to her, trying anything she could think of to keep her awake.

Patty knew from her nurses' training that it is dangerous to fall asleep after an overdose and risk choking on your own vomit. But, by 3 p.m., she needed to get to work.

Maybe I should call and tell them that there's been an emergency, Patty told my mother.

Just go, my mother told Patty. *She'll be fine.*

But she wasn't.

Somehow, Nancy slipped out the back door and staggered toward the train tracks three blocks west. She arrived at about 4:50 p.m., just as the rush hour Chicago and Northwestern commuter train was rumbling south from Kenilworth toward the Wilmette station.

Witnesses would later tell the police that Nancy kept staggering down the tracks, ignoring the train's many whistle blasts. The engineer told police that he slammed on the brakes when he saw that Nancy wasn't moving out of the way, but it was too late. The train skidded right into her, throwing her body into the culvert.

I'm not sure how long it took for my parents to learn that Nancy had been hit. They made their way to the waiting area of Evanston Hospital's emergency room while doctors down the hall took inventory of Nancy's many broken bones and worked to stop the bleeding in her brain. This was the same room where they'd gathered five years earlier after she tried to drown herself in the bathroom. She'd come through then, but such an outcome seemed extremely unlikely now.

An hour passed. The doctor came out to say they were doing all they could but it was not looking promising. My parents knew it was time to rally the troops. They tried calling Mary Kay and me, but we were out buying beer for the party. They dispatched their friends to collect Billy from the grocery store and Patty from the restaurant. Jake and Danny were on a fishing trip in northern Wisconsin. Someone would need to get ahold of them eventually, but that could wait until they knew how all of this would turn out. Lynyrd Skynyrd's "Free Bird" was blasting on the stereo at the grade school graduation party where Molly and her group of friends stood around flirting and chitchatting. Father Hartmann, one of our parish priests, walked across the room, put his hands on Molly's shoulder, and whispered into her ear. *You need to come with me, sweetheart.*

With every minute, hope faded. They said a rosary. *Pray for us sinners, now and at the hour of our death.*

Mary Kay and I had just returned to her apartment when Holmer finally got ahold of us a little after 8 p.m. Nancy was still alive, he said, but just barely. *Hurry.*

Do you think this is it? I asked Mary Kay as we sped north on Sheridan Road. My thoughts were racing, too. What should I wish for? That she survives yet again or that she is finally out of her misery? These last five years had been especially tortuous for Nancy. She seemed so sick, like an end-stage cancer patient growing weaker each day. Each new suicide attempt had taken a little more out of her. We couldn't imagine how she would ever be able to have the kind of life she wanted.

But Holmer never gave up on her. He'd met enough people at his AA meetings who had turned their lives around to believe that recovery is always possible. *It works if you work it,* Holmer would say as he passed out cookies on Christmas Eve to the men and women in the flophouses on Chicago's skid row. In Holmer's world, no one was a lost cause. If these people could get their acts together, his bright, beautiful daughter could, too. *You're so young and talented,* he'd tell her. *You've got so much life ahead of you.*

I wasn't as convinced.

Maybe she doesn't want to be rescued again and again, I thought as we made our way toward the hospital. *Maybe we're being selfish by working so hard to keep her alive when what she wants most of all is to be out of her pain.*

Just after 8:30 p.m., the lead doctor came into the waiting area to let my parents know that there was nothing more they could do. Nancy's injuries were too catastrophic. They were all very sorry. As awful and awkward as it was, someone would need to identify her body. Holmer followed the doctor into the operating room. They asked my mother if she would like to come, too, but she declined.

Mary Kay and I could see Holmer pacing on the hospital lawn with his hands on his head as we drove past the emergency room entrance. As we ran toward him, we could tell by the look in his eyes what he was about to say.

She's gone, he sobbed, then pulled us toward him. We stood under the neon lights, and I could feel my father's chest heaving. *Our little Nanny Goat.*

The sun had just set against a salmon-colored sky. It was going on 9 p.m.

WE ALL HEADED BACK to Greenwood Avenue in a kind of daze. It felt spooky walking into that dark house knowing Nancy was not there and never would be again. I headed to my bedroom, trying not to look down the hall.

Now what? What do we do without Nancy? She'd taken up so much of the energy in our family, it was hard to imagine what life was going to be like without her. I flopped on my bed and stared at the ceiling, trying to make sense of what had just happened.

A few minutes later, Holmer called us all into the living room. He knew that word of Nancy's death would have made its way around the parish by now. The crowd would be descending soon with their bottles of Scotch and store-bought cookies and any other sugary, salty, fatty comfort food they could rustle up in a hurry.

Listen, he said, panting, as he pointed his finger at each of us, like a drill sergeant. *If anyone asks, this was an accident.*

An accident? *Yeah, right,* I thought. *Like anyone is stupid enough to buy that.* How many times had they seen an ambulance in front of our house over the past five years? But Holmer wasn't fooling.

An accident, he said again.

More secrets, more lies, just like when my mother disappeared years earlier. Why couldn't we just tell the damn truth? By hiding what really happened, we'd not only be dismissing Nancy's suffering but fortifying the notion that her mental illness was a choice, one that we should all be ashamed of.

No doubt Holmer was embarrassed that his daughter had killed herself. People always blame the parents. *Why couldn't they have controlled that girl? . . . I heard it was street drugs.*

But there was more to Holmer's cover-up than that. He was also scared that Nancy would be denied a proper Catholic funeral.

In the eyes of the Catholic Church, suicide was considered a sin, and those who killed themselves were destined to burn in hell. Their bodies were declared to be unclean, unworthy of a funeral Mass or burial in a Catholic cemetery. Holmer knew well how cruel the consequences were.

A few years earlier, the fourteen-year-old son of one of his childhood friends hanged himself. Holmer's friend and his wife, daily Mass attendees, were devastated when their parish priest said their son's body would not be permitted inside the church, defiled as it was by the stain of suicide. There could be no funeral Mass, no sprinkling of holy water on the casket, or any kind of final blessing. As Holmer and hundreds of other mourners filled the pews for a simple memorial service, the casket with the dead boy's body idled in a hearse parked down the block. Holmer didn't want poor Nancy's battered body idling in the back of any hearse.

Still, an accident? If we objected to Holmer's command that we hide the truth, there was no time for debate about it or questions. And there certainly wasn't time for a check-in to see how we were all feeling about Nancy and the gruesome way she had just died. Only more orders: *Straighten up this house! Get all these damn shoes off the front porch. Do we have enough ice?*

Sure enough, within minutes of our arrival back home, the good people of St. Francis Xavier started to swarm. By 10 p.m., our house was buzzing with people, whispering at first and awkwardly hugging. Then out came the cigarettes and the bottles of booze. Jack Daniel's. Tanqueray gin. Of course, Jameson. Pretty soon, the joint was jumpin'.

Nothing captivates a bunch of Irish people more than a sad story and a stiff drink. We offered them plenty of both. The house was filling up fast. We would need to turn on our charm, put on our best party faces, and make these folks feel welcome.

Holmer weaved through the crowd with his mug of coffee, hugging and wiping away his tears with his signature fashion statement: a big red bandanna that he always kept in his back pocket. My mother sat in one of the blue velvet living room chairs, looking dazed. She nodded between sips of her martini just as she had that Thanksgiving afternoon so many years earlier when she was home on a three-hour pass.

More friends came pouring into the kitchen door. Neighbors. Relatives. *Oh, you poor kid,* one of my parents' boozy dinner club pals said as she pulled me toward her ample bosom, calling me Nancy by mistake. *Oh, God, I'm sorry,* she said. *I'm SO sorry.* Still others arrived by the side door.

We started in with stories about Nancy. It made us happy to talk about her, to keep her with us a while longer. The last five years had been such a mess. It was a relief to think about her before she got so sick.

What a whiz she was at the keyboard, someone said. *She loved those bluesy ballads,* said another. *And cute? Oh, she was so cute. That button nose.*

More people. More food. More booze. *Remember the time she had two dates to the same dance without either guy knowing about the other?* The living room was jammed, and the playroom was starting to get crowded, too.

Here you go, Meg, someone said, handing me another beer.

My turn now. *This story may have been embellished over the years,* I told them, *but I'll tell it anyway.*

Years ago, my mother's uncle, a man of about fifty, died suddenly of a heart attack. My mother wanted to go to the wake to pay her respects, but she couldn't find a babysitter. So, she bundled us up and lugged us along to the funeral home. We inched along with the line of mourners and eventually made our way to the casket, where the grieving widow stood. Nancy, who was no more than four years old, grabbed the side of the wooden box, pulled herself up on her tiptoes, and gazed at the corpse.

Oh well, little Nancy said, shrugging at the widow. *We all have to go sometime.*

Everyone roared.

As the house heated up, the din grew louder. I found myself climbing upstairs to sneak into Nancy's room. I hadn't seen her dead body at the hospital. None of us had, except Holmer. Even with a house full of mourners, it was hard to believe that Nancy was really gone, that she wouldn't just walk in the back door at any minute, making a mess in the kitchen, telling me to go fetch her cigarettes. *How do we know she's not really on her way to join a rock band in California?* Mary Kay wondered.

As I walked into Nancy's bedroom, I could see that the covers on her canopy bed had been pulled back like she'd been in a hurry to get somewhere. Or was that just my imagination, now that I knew how the story ended? Her pillow was still dented where her head had been just a few hours before. Her bathrobe lay crumpled in the corner. I leaned down and picked it up, taking in a big whiff, a familiar blend of Kool cigarettes and Noxzema face cream. That's when I saw her alarm clock, the cord pulled from the socket.

4:17.

Had she done that on purpose? I was looking for clues, grasping for a tidy story line, a way to make sense of all of this. Was this her one last act before stumbling toward the train tracks, a message, a metaphor? Did she want us to know that time had stopped for her? *So long, suckers.*

We all have to go sometime.

What was the matter with me? Maybe the beer was making me giddy.

I plopped down on the gold velvet armchair across from Nancy's bed and felt my shoulders start to shake. *She's gone,* I thought. *Gone forever. Never coming back.* After a few deep breaths to steady myself, I noticed something strange. My whole body was starting to relax so that I could feel the tension releasing from every muscle from the top of my head down to my toes. I felt light, like a cloud that could float away, breezy, fluffy, and free.

This reaction sounds crazy, I know. Nancy was dead. I would never see her again. I felt like I should be sobbing, and I was confused about why I wasn't. But for the last several years, I had been terrified of her. She made all our lives miserable. No one wanted to hear that, but it was true. And this is also true: She was the most miserable of us all. Each day seemed worse than the last for her. Who would want to keep living like that? The fact is, I was relieved she was gone, for my sake and hers. And now a houseful of guests were downstairs, waiting to cheer me up and comfort me, the sad, grieving little sister.

Only I wasn't really grieving, at least not in a way they expected me to be or in a way that I understood.

IT RAINED SO HARD that night that our basement flooded for the first time in the fifteen years that we lived there. Holmer spent most of the next day down there mopping up the mess while my mother went from closet to closet looking for outfits that each of us could wear to the wake and funeral. We also needed to figure out a way to get Jake and Danny home from their fishing trip in northern Wisconsin. Holmer didn't think Jake should be driving for seven hours after hearing such terrible news. So my parents booked a one-way ticket for Mary Kay to fly up there so that she could help Jake drive Danny and his friends back home.

People kept stopping by to drop off casseroles and coffee cakes until both refrigerators and freezers were full. Everything was happening so fast. We had no time to let this sink in.

The wake was set for the next day, a Sunday. The funeral would be the day after that. We kicked into showtime mode. That was fine with me. It was easier to worry about what shoes matched which dress than to sit around and reflect on the fact that our sister was dead.

As it turned out, that Sunday was also Father's Day, typically reserved for breakfast in bed, rounds of golf, cheesy greeting cards, and new ties. I couldn't imagine a sadder contrast for Holmer than to have to spend the day standing next to his daughter's casket.

I had written him a cheeky poem on Friday afternoon, just forty-eight hours earlier, before any of this happened, titled "An Ode to Our Non-Drinking Dad" to celebrate his sobriety, now two years strong. As the mourners began streaming into the parking lot, I handed Holmer a copy, hoping it might cheer him up.

Sometimes you're a brat,
Sometimes you're a fink.
But we're proud of you, Dad
Cuz you don't drink.

He read a few stanzas, folded it up, and tucked it into his suit coat pocket. *Thanks, kid,* he said, his voice catching.

Nancy's closed casket spared us from having to stare at her dead body, but it also served as a reminder of how she died, that she'd been too mangled to be put on display.

The line at the funeral home snaked into the hall and out the door. Holmer, standing next to my mother, worked the room like Johnny Carson, kissing the ladies, hugging the men, and telling his funny stories just quickly enough to keep the people moving along. Technically, the mourners were there to comfort us, but we—or at least I—felt it should be the other way around. I felt guilty about putting our friends and relatives in such an awkward position, to have to come to us under these ugly circumstances, on Father's Day no less. *Let's keep this breezy,* I thought.

The seven of us surviving siblings lined up beside our parents like a cheerleading squad waiting for the players to take the field. *Soggy Lips Trio alert,* I leaned over and whispered to Patty as our three wrinkled old aunts waddled through the door.

The room seemed strangely festive on this sunny Sunday afternoon in June, the air smelling of peonies, the near-solstice sunlight streaming into the lobby, promising carefree days ahead, swinging on the hammock, splashing on the shore. With friends and relatives coming in from out of town, our gathering felt more like a wedding reception. I half expected to hear Bee Gees music being piped into the background. So, it was not entirely surprising when my friend Joan got a call a few days later from a guy saying, *I don't know if you remember me, but we met at the Nancy Kissinger wake,* as if it were a Sigma Nu kegger.

But as the night wore on and the guests began to peel away, it was clear that we would soon have to acknowledge that this indeed was not a frat party but a wake for our dead sister, a dead sister who had killed herself. Just as the gathering was about to end, a busload of nuns from our high school showed up to say the rosary. One old nun, who taught us math, pulled Mary Kay aside, pointed at Nancy's casket, and whispered, *She's going to hell, you know.*

Nancy had sinned. She would burn for eternity. There would be no peace for her. What if the bishop found out that Nancy killed herself? Would he call off the Mass? Would her body have to idle in the back of the hearse after all? No one slept well that night.

The next morning, we shuffled nervously into the vestibule of St. Francis, and as the doors to the church swung open, I could see my mother's shoulders slump with relief. There, inside, was a standing-room-only crowd and not just one but three priests at the altar ready to say the funeral Mass. The pallbearers, uncles, cousins, and Nancy's loyal science fair pal Ellen, rolled the casket down the aisle. One hurdle crossed. One more to go. Having her body consecrated for burial was one thing. Having it put into the ground would be another.

After the mass, we formed a convoy and drove ninety minutes north up to Holy Cross Cemetery in Milwaukee, where my mother's family had the deeds to several burial plots. Never skilled navigators, several of us got lost on the way. We drove around for more than half an hour before spotting Holmer marching back and forth in the middle of the road, frantically flagging us down.

Goddamn it, Holmer said, directing us toward the grave. *Can't this fucking family do anything right?*

The priest looked at his watch and grimaced as we huddled by the casket so he could give the final blessing.

Ashes to ashes, dust to dust, the priest said, sprinkling the casket with holy water. Then we each took a flower and tossed it into the hole. As we headed back to the cars, on our way to a German restaurant for long-awaited steins of cold beer, we heard a slight beep. And then another. And another. *Beep. Beep. Beeeeeeep.* We turned around to see a backhoe winching Nancy's casket out of the ground. *Nancy, rising from the tomb on the third day, just like Jesus himself!*

The truth was a lot less Holy Bible and a lot more holy shit. The gravediggers had gone on strike, and the substitute crew mistakenly put her casket in the wrong spot. They would have to turn over a new plot and bury her all over again. It could take an hour or more.

Fuck it, Holmer said, and we turned back around to head to the restaurant. As we pulled away, we could see Nancy's casket hanging on the crane, swinging slightly.

Wait, Mary Kay said, pressing her nose against the car window for a better view. *Is she waving to us?*

A part of me wanted to think that was exactly what she was doing, that this was another sign from Nancy, like unplugging her bedroom clock. I wanted to believe that Nancy was punking us from the great beyond. Was Nancy trying to get one more rise out of us, the sneaky little way she used to stick her tongue out at me at the dinner table when Holmer and my mother had their backs turned?

Maybe Nancy thought that we'd be better off without her. I hoped we'd be better now, too. Not that I ever wished for her to die. But now that Nancy was dead, I hoped she was at peace and we could find some, too.

Little did I know how wrong I'd be.

THREE DAYS LATER, I sat on the limestone steps of our front porch, nervously picking petals off the potted hot-pink geraniums and listening for the newspaper delivery truck to come clattering down our redbrick street. The *Wilmette Life* would be showing up any minute now, and I wasn't about to let my poor mother see what was in it. Hadn't she been through enough?

When the newspaper arrived, I opened it and quickly found what I was looking for—the three-paragraph story about my sister on the left-hand side of the page: WOMAN DIES AFTER BEING HIT BY TRAIN.

I ripped the story out and stuffed it into my pocket. The budding journalist in me knew why it was important to report this story. That's our job. We record history, disturbing as it may be. But I also knew that my mother didn't need to read it.

While she was up in the attic taking a nap, I ducked into my bedroom and slid the clipping into the back of my dresser drawer, underneath my socks and underwear. *My new little secret hiding place.*

I may have spared my mother the anguish of reading in black and white about how the train slammed into Nancy. But I couldn't protect her from her own inevitable crash and burn.

We started finding my mother's empty gin bottles at the bottom of the clothes hamper that summer. By the following spring, she was spending most of her time napping in the attic. That's where Holmer found her one afternoon curled on the bed with her back facing the door. He called out to her, but she didn't answer. So, he ran to her side and rolled her over.

Her body was cold.

8

A Hard Molt

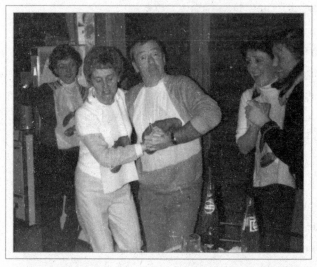

Lobster night (note the Pepsi bottles on the table where the martini glasses once were). Patty, my mother, Holmer, me, and Molly. Greenwood Avenue, Wilmette, Illinois, 1978.

Holmer called me the day before my college graduation to warn me. He and the rest of my family might not make it to the ceremony. No one could be sure when my mother was going to be released from alcohol rehab.

Don't hold your breath, he said.

It had been a few weeks since Holmer discovered my mother passed out on the bed up in the attic. She swore that she was not trying to kill herself that day. She just lost track of how much she had to drink. That's all. Vodka and sleeping pills don't mix well.

Ever since Nancy died eleven months earlier, my mother was quick to reach for the bottle. A nip of vodka in the morning while doing the laundry, a swig of gin as she got dinner going. Just like in her high school days, alcohol helped her to relax. Now she added a new feature to her repertoire: A glass or two (or three) of white wine in the middle of the night helped dull the pain when her thoughts turned to Nancy stumbling toward the tracks. Patty and I could hear our mother walking up and down the stairs at all hours.

Good thing you got to her when you did, the doctor told Holmer after he rushed her to the hospital. *A few more minutes, and you might have been planning another funeral.*

Once my mother was stabilized, the doctor sent her to the alcohol rehab unit to detox. My academic career would end as it had begun sixteen years earlier—with my mother in the hospital and my stomach in knots. Most likely, she would stay for two weeks, but it would depend on how well she responded to treatment. Holmer had been "clean and sober" for three years now and he was eager to share the lessons he'd learned at his AA meetings about the value of sobriety.

"Learning to turn it over to God!!!" he wrote in the margins of his AA book. "Alcohol was the key thing in my life. I depended on it."

No one would blame him if he took a swig or two to steady his nerves around the time that Nancy died. But he never did, not even once. I figured if Holmer could give up booze, anyone could, even my mother.

"My worst day sober is far better than the best day as an alcoholic," he wrote in the margins of his AA book. "I need to learn to <u>SURRENDER!!!!</u>"

Holmer was a scrapper and a man of enthusiasms, unafraid to show his emotions. He knew you sometimes had to use sharp elbows and sacrifice comfort to accomplish your goals. But my mother played life closer to the vest. With her Jane Austen–like sensibilities and country club manners, she was more private and discerning, less inclined to herd mentality. We'd have to wait and see if AA's program of slogan-chanting and confessionals would work for her.

As my college friends' families began to gather for the graduation festivities, I sat on the sorority's front porch swing, feeling lonely and disappointed and more than a little sorry for myself. *Look at them parading around campus in their black caps and graduation gowns, slapping high fives and hugging.*

I could feel my face getting warmer.

Of course my family wasn't going to make it to my graduation, I thought as I pumped my legs, and the big wooden swing moved back and forth. *Nancy's dead, and now my mother is drinking herself to death. What a fucking bunch of losers we're all turning out to be.*

My legs were pushing harder now, and the swing started to squeak. I thought about Flip the Bird, our family's pet canary, and how he used to swing like this in his cage just before all his feathers fell out.

Each year, at about this time, Flip would stop singing, and some days, he'd just lie on his side on the bottom of his cage, staring into space. We worried that he was dead. *No, no,* my mother would assure us. *He'll be fine again in no time. He's just having a hard molt.*

We all had a hard molt the year that Nancy died. We just didn't know what to do about it. On Tuesday, June 20, 1978, the day after Nancy's funeral, it was back to business as usual on Greenwood Avenue. Work. Laundry. Wiffle ball games. Making dinner. *Will somebody please mow that damn lawn?*

We simply went back to our old routines with no therapy or family discussions. None. I don't remember talking at any length about Nancy's death to anyone that summer—not to my friends, not to my parents, not to Patty, my roommate and Tiger Pit pal, not even to Mary Kay, who helped me land a summer job as a receptionist at her little marketing firm. We just waited for time to heal us, hoping that nature would restore our spirits the way it had Flip's feathers.

Although I was staying at Mary Kay's apartment a few nights each week, I now thought it was important for me to be at home more, to add to the clatter so my parents felt less lonely. Friends came by as they always did, but I don't remember anybody asking us about Nancy or how we were getting along. They probably thought it would be too painful for us if they mentioned her.

Of course, we were thinking about her hundreds of times a day, especially each time we passed her bedroom and saw her clothes still hanging on the side of her chair or her guitar leaning against the wall.

The only sustained reference to her was a subtle change in our nightly dinnertime blessing. Now, instead of saying, "Eternal rest grant unto *him,* O Lord," as a shout-out to our long-dead uncle, Jack, we switched the third-person pronoun to "them." Nancy was in our prayers but not in our conversations. Our dinner discussions were mostly nonsense, dialogue from old TV shows, plans for the week or neighborhood gossip, anything but Nancy.

My old social life didn't appeal to me much that summer. Most nights, I stayed in, slipping into my pajamas after dinner and watching baseball. I kept track of the batters' balls and strikes count with a clicker like the kind the umpires use. Hanging on every pitch is a great way to tune out reality.

In late August, I returned to campus for my senior year and threw myself into my job as school newspaper editor, glad for the distraction. I much preferred to take on the new university president's power struggles with the tenured faculty and the alcohol-induced misadventures of our hapless 0–9 football team than to let my mind wander. Journalism was providing me with a perfect escape. If I could focus on the tensions of the stories I was working on, I wouldn't have to think about the drama at home.

But all that unprocessed grief was starting to express itself in other ways. When I wasn't busy, I was quick to break into tears or to down a bottle of beer. I couldn't figure out how life could just keep chugging along as normal when mine had been shattered. I started to resent the thrum of everyday life, the routines and the rituals at the sorority house that I once found charming, even comforting or amusing. Even the smallest things seemed to be bugging me now, especially the ridiculous way my sorority sisters got so whipped up about rush, sobbing when someone they hoped would pledge joined another house. It all seemed so petty and inconsequential. *People are dying, and this is what you are crying about?*

A few weeks into the semester, I ran out of a class on Hemingway in tears when the professor blithely described how the author had blown his brains out with one of his hunting rifles. Later that month, I cut my own hair after too many beers. A few weeks after that, I called my parents at 1:30 a.m., crying that my stomach hurt, when, really, I was worried about them. Of course, I never said that to them. I didn't want them to worry that I was worried.

My reckless behavior was not going unnoticed in the sorority house. I got drunk at the homecoming football game and made a spectacle of myself by dancing with the team mascot (a *tiger!*) on the fifty-yard line at halftime. Members of my sorority's governing board summoned me before them the following week to warn me that I was in danger of losing my membership for engaging in "behavior unbecoming of a Kappa Alpha Theta." What did I have to say for myself? Not much. I was embarrassed, of course. What I wanted to say was, *Cut me some slack, you prissy old hags. My sister jumped in front of a goddamn train and my mother is a hot fucking mess.* Instead, I nodded and said I was sorry. I needed a shoulder to cry on, not a stern lecture about etiquette. This would have been a great opportunity for someone to suggest grief counseling or for me to see a doctor. Again, it didn't happen.

At Thanksgiving, I noticed how thin my mother was. By Christmas, she looked even worse.

At least she's not suffering anymore, my mother muttered as she stood at the sink doing dishes that Christmas night. We were all nervous about how to get through those first holidays without Nancy. The movie *It's a Wonderful Life* was showing on TV around the clock, now that its copyright had expired, and we got obsessed with its plot—a foiled suicide attempt. "No man is a failure who has friends," the guardian angel Clarence tells George Bailey. Why didn't we think of that? Where was Nancy's guardian angel? My mother bought too many presents. Holmer made too much food. We all laughed a little too hard, acted a little too silly, and all, except Holmer, drank a little too much, hoping the excess would fill the space Nancy left. If we acted like we were having fun, maybe it would come true.

For the first time since Nancy died, my mother was starting to talk about her. She said she didn't cry at Nancy's funeral, not because she wasn't sad. She just couldn't summon the tears. *I think I'm just so relieved that she's not in pain anymore.* I was grateful that my mother was talking about her reaction to Nancy's death, sad as it was. This was progress. But our discussion didn't go any further than that. She never said, *How are you doing?* Not wanting to add to her worries, I refrained from disclosing my true feelings, whatever those were. I wasn't really sure.

Most of us weren't interested in examining our feelings. Now that we had come up with the party line—*She's much better off now*—we were looking for an easy way to move on. The two exceptions would be Jake, the philosopher, who was always willing to discuss what happened and posit why, and Danny, who was fifteen and made no secret of the fact that he was angry with Nancy. Very angry. And embarrassed. He said he thought suicide was a "coward's way out" and told people that Nancy had been killed in a car crash. I dismissed Danny's behavior as a by-product of being young and immature. *He'll see in time,* I thought.

By late winter, it was clear to us all that my mother's drinking had gotten out of control. She used to call Patty and me at our respective schools on Sunday afternoons to catch us up on the latest news: *Billy was accepted at Vanderbilt and Georgetown. Danny and his friends are going skiing this weekend. Molly's basketball team won their game on Friday. That's four in a row.* But now, after we had hung up, she would call back an hour later and repeat everything. *Yeah, I know, Mom,* I would say sharply. *You already told me that. Don't you remember?*

I called Patty. *Mom's losing it.* I had no patience for any more drama.

My mother had gotten a job that winter, something she had not had since she was first married. Some of her friends sold real estate or worked at tony little boutiques as a way to pass the time. But we needed the cash. With Patty and me in college and three more kids to follow, money was even tighter.

My mother got a job as a cashier at a liquor store (a dangerous choice) not far from home, but she couldn't figure out how to give proper change, so, after a week, they fired her. Next, she tried our local hardware store, with the same result. *Wow,* I thought when I heard the news. *Talk about bottoming out. The debutante with the genius IQ gets shitcanned from a liquor store.* Then, she stopped cooking dinner for the family and took to the attic each afternoon.

By now, I was furious with her. We needed a mother, goddamn it, someone to be our rock, to ask us how we were dealing with Nancy's death, to listen to our fears, and give us encouragement. *At a bare minimum, make dinner for these kids, for Christ's sake,* I thought.

When I went home for spring break, I was appalled to see Molly and Danny and Billy making their own meals. Holmer cooked when he wasn't traveling for work. Otherwise, the three youngest kids, now all in high school, were on their own. Of course, they were capable of feeding themselves. Plenty of teenagers are pressed into tougher duty than microwaving lasagna, but I felt sad for my younger siblings, who didn't have the kind of luxury I had growing up—hearing my mother ring the big brass dinner bell each night. We would scramble to the table every night at 6:30 sharp to find mounds of food waiting for us.

I made a cardboard sign and put it around Molly's neck reading, "Please feed me." I hoped my attempt at humor, however mean-spirited I now see it as, would shake some sense of duty into my mother.

It didn't. In fact, she was getting worse.

So, I wasn't that surprised when Holmer called me in early May to tell me what had happened up in the attic and how my mother was now finally, thank God, going to get help for her drinking. If she'd been diagnosed with cancer or had suffered a heart attack, I'm sure I would have left school right away and gone home to visit her. At the very least, I would have called her and told her how sorry I was that she was not well. I would be worried sick, praying for her and asking my friends to do the same. But this was her mental illness, something many of us at that time considered a weakness in her character, real "Days of Wine and Roses" shit. If only she could be stronger. I kept my distance and my mouth shut.

By late evening on the night before my college graduation, the campus was crawling with guests. Boz Scaggs's "Lido Shuffle" was blaring through the sorority house as I started to make my way down the front lawn. And that's when I saw them. The family station wagon pulled up to the Theta house, and there they were. My parents and six remaining siblings spilled out of the station wagon, a Kissinger family clown car. Beat up and bedraggled as they were, I had never seen such a welcome sight.

My family made it to my graduation after all. My mother was released from the hospital not long after Holmer's phone call to me. *Come with me,* I said, parading them around campus, stopping to pose for pictures, and introducing them to everyone. *Here they are!*

My mother still looked shaky, but she was doing her best to put on a good show.

Nice going, kid, she said when we met up after the ceremony.

On the way home, Holmer laughed at how broadly the university president smiled as he handed me my diploma. I had tormented that poor man with my newspaper stories and editorials.

He looked damn glad to be getting rid of you.

MARY KAY HAD ANNOUNCED earlier that spring that she was treating me to a two-week trip to Ireland to celebrate my graduation. *I would have settled for a cheap watch or a piece of luggage,* I told her jokingly, stunned at her largesse. She had spent the last month planning it all, from the airline tickets to the hotels and car rental. I just had to show up. After the year we had been through, we were hungry for adventure, and we could not imagine anywhere as stirring as Ireland. It had all we needed—rocky coastlines, quaint shops, and, of course, Guinness. Grandma had brainwashed us all into thinking that there was no land as magical or people as charming.

At the last minute, my mother suggested that we take Patty, too. Her treat. Patty, who had always been thin, was looking increasingly pale and worn down since Nancy died. *I should have stayed home that day,* she said more than once. My mother was worried about Patty. *She could use a jolly escapade,* my mother said.

The three of us took off for Shannon the week after my graduation.

We traipsed through the Dingle Peninsula, on to Limerick and Dublin, then up to county Meath where John Lynch, our great-grandfather, was born. The house where he was raised had been converted to a pigsty.

Not surprised, said Mary Kay as we tried peering through the shit-caked windows. *Explains a lot.*

He might have gotten a laugh at the notion of his great-granddaughters romanticizing the country that failed him and his family so miserably. Like so many Irish of that era, the Lynches were forced to leave home if they were to survive. The land, stunningly beautiful as it was to us now, was harsh and unforgiving in those days, crops failing year after year.

I wondered what he would think of us and our "troubles," the way Nancy and the rest of us put up such a fuss when we had so much—a comfortable home, good food on the table, central heating, indoor plumbing. *Bellyachers,* I imagine he might have said.

Nancy thought too much, I said to Patty and Mary Kay as we sat sipping our Guinness one night.

Well, that's never been my problem, Mary Kay said, and we all took another swig.

Three days after we got back, I was off to upstate New York, thrilled at the chance to work as a general assignment reporter on the *Watertown Daily Times.*

OUR CAR STARTED SHAKING just west of Elkhart, Indiana. Then the engine light popped on, and we knew we were not going to be able to go any farther without getting this checked out.

Well, shit, I said, turning into the nearest auto repair shop.

My mother, three weeks out of alcohol rehab, and Billy, who was bound for his freshman year at the University of Michigan, were driving me out to Watertown. We were toting a U-Haul with Grandma's dresser, Nancy's old red ski jacket, a mattress, and a few cardboard boxes that I would later use as a coffee table. The mechanic glanced under the hood and told us we needed a new transmission part. He would have to order one from the next town over.

It's gonna be a while, the man said.

My mother shot a little glance toward town and said she would wait at the service station with the car, and why don't Billy and I go see the sights?

That should take about ten minutes, I said, looking around, snapping my fingers the way Holmer always did when he was antsy. It was 9 a.m., and we had another 630 miles to go.

Indeed, we didn't find much to hold our interest in town. When Billy and I got back to the car, about a half an hour later, our mother was gone.

She went that way, the mechanic said, pointing back toward town.

I knew exactly where to find her.

This way, I told Billy, marching toward the first bar we saw. Sure enough, there was my mother, sipping a martini. It was 9:45 a.m.

Ooops, she said and smiled when I bolted through the door. I wanted to slap her. My whole body was shaking. How dare she, after the hell she just put us all through! She could have died up in that attic. And then what? Leave Holmer a widower to raise these kids? I prayed every day that my mother would find the strength and the courage to put down the god-damn vodka bottle and be a grown-up. But, no. She can't control herself now and, truth be told, she never could.

You are pathetic, I thought, staring back at her. *You're a weak, spineless, selfish woman.*

So much for those two weeks in rehab and all the anxiety we felt wondering if she would be able to quit drinking once and for all. *There's your answer,* I thought. *Right there in that fucking martini glass.*

In a battle between the well-being of her family and her precious alcohol, my mother chose to drink.

A little while later, we were back on the road, but I was so angry I could barely speak. My new life in Watertown could not come fast enough.

John Johnson, my new boss, had warned me that this might not be my idea of a dream job when he offered me the position the previous November.

"I have only one caveat which I outline only because I consider you a good friend," he wrote. He and I became pals earlier that fall when he came to campus for a few weeks to serve as the advisor for *The DePauw,* the campus newspaper that I edited. He liked my spunk, and I liked his seemingly endless enthusiasm for a good scoop. "Watertown, while it has 30,000 people, can be a socially stifling place. In short, there are not many eligible males floating about."

While I appreciated his concern, I wasn't hunting for a husband. I was hungry for bylines.

Despite my enthusiasm for the job, I was so miserable by the second day, I thought about bolting for home. I'd never lived on my own, and I had no idea how to budget anything—my time, my energy, especially my money. I didn't know how to cook, much less balance a checkbook. My parents were too frazzled to teach us these life skills, which, frankly, they weren't so good at either.

I knew nothing about getting by on my own. I had never even spent a night alone. Just before leaving me that Saturday morning, my parents gave me a check for two hundred dollars and a twenty-dollar bill to get me through the weekend. I had no credit cards. This was before ATMs, and the only way to get money was at a bank, and they were closed on weekends.

In my zeal to clean my new apartment, I spent all but $1.85 on a toilet brush, Windex, Comet, and a few houseplants. When I got back from the store, I realized to my horror that my refrigerator was empty. So was the pantry. I would have to get by for the next forty-plus hours on the only thing I could think of that cost under two bucks—a Whopper Jr., small fries, and a Diet Coke. My new apartment was clean now that I'd scrubbed the bejeezus out of it, but, by Sunday night, I was feeling woozy.

I started my professional journalism career the next day with a blinding headache and a growling stomach filled with butterflies. *I've made a terrible mistake,* I told my mother when I called home sobbing later that week. My anger at her Elkhart, Indiana, morning martini had subsided. I had more urgent matters in mind. *They're having me writing wedding announcements and obituaries and some stupid column about what happened here on this date in history. Nothing happens here! I'm in the middle of nowhere.* I'd imagined a much more glamorous life as a young reporter living in New York. Of course, this was northern New York. If I'd bothered to consult a map more thoroughly, I would have realized that New York City was seven hours away by car. *Please come back and bring me home.* Two days later, my mother sent me this letter:

June 28, 1979

Hello, old girl,

I miss you like crazy. We all do. I know it's a tough time for you right now. You just got what you wanted and now you are not so sure that you're going to be happy, but you just have to give it some time. Probably by the time you get this letter, you will have made about ten new friends like you always do. Good that you got your apartment straightened out and got some plants. They can be your friends for a while.

My mother, struggling to find a way to stay sober, was summoning all her maternal instincts to come to my rescue. Her words were so warm and cheerful, I couldn't help but feel encouraged. She was affirming and comforting to me on paper in ways that she could not manage to be in the flesh.

She must have been worried sick about me. Maybe she thought that I was falling apart, too. One kid of hers after another was growing up and melting down. If she was scared, she did not show it. She didn't scold me for being such a jackass and making poor spending choices. She acknowledged my feelings, accentuated the positive, and subtly urged me to do the same. *Maybe she's right,* I thought.

A few weeks later, Holmer came to visit. He claimed he was passing by Watertown on his way back to Wilmette from New York City, but I'm pretty sure my mother sent him to check up on me. Holmer came to visit again a few months later, and we went cross-country skiing, something neither of us had any idea how to do. We had done plenty of downhill skiing, but no cross-country.

Little steps! Holmer kept shouting to me as we tried to maneuver our way through the forest without breaking our necks. This, of course, is the opposite of how you cross-country ski. But, as I picked myself up again and again, I appreciated that Holmer had gone out of his way to come see me, that I was important enough to him to notice that I was struggling. Just like that day at the eye doctor with my mother many years earlier, this adventure with Holmer felt like stolen time, a luxury.

We didn't talk about Nancy or my mother's battles. Our conversation was mostly banter, silliness about Watertown, which he called *Watergoose*. Holmer was tickled to learn that I was already stirring things up with my newspaper stories, making a name for myself as a rabble-rouser. A critical review I wrote of a Slim Whitman concert had upset so many readers that a local radio host challenged me to an arm wrestling contest, and I accepted. We laughed about my battles with the officious public information officer at Fort Drum, the nearby army base who once referred to me as a "bumpy-chested reporter," and how I managed to get a few scoops already. Holmer still was not prepared to talk about feelings—his or mine. He was there to "jolly me up," give me a shot of confidence.

But the unspoken message of his visits was clear: I wasn't Nancy. I was different. Yes, I was emotional, and I felt things intensely. But that didn't mean I was destined to end up like she did. If I could take on these authority figures, challenge the status quo, arm wrestle a radio announcer, and stand up to a misogynistic army officer, I could get past a "case of the blues."

Keep chugging, Muggs, Holmer said to me that day in the woods. He was probably talking about my skiing, but I chose a broader interpretation.

My mother was right about me feeling better but she was wrong about me making ten new friends in Watertown. I did make a few, including one who changed my life. He may have even saved it. Larry Boynton was the rarest of species, an eligible Watertown male.

GREAT VIEW AHEAD JUST *over these rocks!* Larry shouted as I trudged behind him, feeling like my lungs might explode. Smoking a pack of cigarettes a day does not help prepare you to hike the Adirondack Mountains or any of the other adventures he was dragging me to. I should have known that he was up to something. He was always tricking me into things like this. We were inching our way up New Hampshire's Mount Washington on a brilliant September morning, a feat so demanding that they sold bumper stickers in the gift shop exclaiming: THIS CAR CLIMBED MT. WASHINGTON.

I met Larry on my first day at the newspaper. He was a reporter, like me, but assigned to one of the many bureaus that the paper manned across the northern fifth of the state. He covered Carthage, a manufacturing and mill town about twenty miles east of Watertown that also had seen better days. His good pal Bob Diddlebock, a Philadelphia native gruff enough to not take shit from anyone about his funny last name, worked as a copy editor at the newspaper and lived in the apartment above mine just a few blocks from the newsroom.

Larry and Bob used to watch baseball games on Bob's grainy Panasonic and roll their empty cans of Genesee beer down the building's hallway steps. I walked up there under the guise of complaining about the noise one Saturday afternoon shortly after moving in and ended up popping open a few cold ones with them. I think they were impressed that I could name most of the batters in the starting lineup of Pops Stargell's "We Are Family" Pittsburgh Pirates. By the Fourth of July, the three of us were scalloping the bars of Alexandria Bay, square-dancing at Johnny Scanlon's Green Acres Inn just outside the tiny town of Harrisville, and navigating the twisty back roads of northern New York in my new lemon-yellow 1979 Toyota Corolla. Three amigos. After a few pitchers of beer, Bob and Larry would hang their heads out of the windows like a couple of rabid hound dogs while I tried to switch into fifth gear without burning out the clutch.

Bob, boisterous and brilliant, had a girlfriend, but Larry, shy and sometimes off-putting, was single, as near as I could tell. He was cute, with thick blond hair, broad shoulders, brilliant blue eyes, and a biting sense of humor. What he lacked in warmth, he made up for in an adventurous spirit. Larry frequently asked me to go skiing or hiking or fishing with him. Even after a few months, I couldn't tell if he had romantic feelings for me. I hadn't had the best track record with boyfriends. Either I liked them too much or vice versa. Since Nancy died, I was too busy and distracted to even try for a meaningful relationship. *There's a guy here who's really cute, but I'm not sure if he's interested in me romantically,* I told my mother on the phone one night. *How do I know if he likes me?* She didn't hesitate.

Get him drunk, my mother said. *That'll shake things loose.* So, I did, and it did.

After Larry and I started dating, I quit smoking cigarettes, figuring I'd need all the lung power I could muster to keep up with him. He squired me around northern New York, lugging me up one Adirondack mountain after another, hauling me to cheese and bologna factories, taking me bullhead fishing (where I caught a pair of wire cutters) and cross-country skiing along the Tug Hill Plateau. He brought me gladiolas, mums, and clumps of roses that smelled faintly of formaldehyde. (I later learned that was because they were recycled, bound for the dumpster of his friend's funeral home.) As frustrating as it was to try to understand his emotions, I was hooked.

When we first started dating, Larry was renting a room from a lady who ran a beauty parlor, and the place smelled like rotten eggs. Then he moved in with the chief of our copy desk, into a 150-year-old woodframed house in the country, heated only by a woodstove in the living room. If you put a glass of water by the bed on some winter nights when the thermometer dipped to twenty below or more, you would wake up the next morning to find a solid block of ice. I'd never known anyone as eccentric as Larry, so full of surprises.

Occasionally, Larry took me along on his reporting adventures. He wrote mainly about agriculture, and so I got to inspect maple syrup operations, dairies, and llama farms, and snicker as a goat ate his notebook. This was all foreign territory for a city girl like me. Larry had his own garden on a plot of land his friend the undertaker owned in the tiny town of Denmark. He called it his Danish garden and taught me how to weed his rows of beans, broccoli, kohlrabi, and carrots. All the vegetables that I ate growing up came frozen, in a can, or wrapped in cellophane on Styrofoam trays. Larry's fresh tomatoes were so sweet, my knees buckled the first time I tasted one.

He made salsa, baked pies, and knit his own scarves. Larry introduced me to a whole new world I never knew existed—fresh food, fresh air, stunning mountain views, the thrill of waking up in a tent as the sun rises and watching an eagle swoop by.

I quickly figured out that Larry was someone I could count on to keep me safe. Outings with him were as calibrated as a NASA space mission. He spent hours planning. Before each of our skiing or hiking trips, Larry packed lunches with just the right balance of sandwiches, fruit, and cookies. He studied the map and always made sure we had sunscreen.

Kissinger adventures were more seat-of-the-pants affairs. Holmer would throw suitcases on top of our station wagon with no thought to how they would best fit, then drape a tarp over the top, and try to tie everything down with rope. More than once, we watched the suitcases roll down the highway like tumbleweeds.

There goes another one! Patty or Billy or I would shout from the rear of the station wagon.

Not long after we started dating, Larry invited me to spend Thanksgiving with his family at their house in the woods outside of Albany, overlooking the Helderberg Escarpment. I felt like I had just walked onto the set of *Father Knows Best*. The rooms were tastefully decorated with his mother's pastel paintings, needlepointed pillows, and family antiques, including a grandfather clock and a Hitchcock chair that predated the Revolutionary War. Serenaded by classical music, we ate off the bone china plates that his great-great-grandfather, a sea captain, had brought back to New England 150 years earlier. The monogrammed cloth napkins were kept in silver rings, also monogrammed. After dinner, we repaired to the living room to watch hours of home movies.

I couldn't take my eyes off the screen. Larry's father (Princeton, Class of '39) and his mother (Smith College, Class of '40) seemed to beam in every frame as Larry and his two younger sisters blew out their birthday candles, marched around in homemade Halloween costumes, and splashed along the shore of their cottage in Lake George. They all looked like little movie stars to me with their straight white teeth. They barreled down the ski slopes of Vermont in their Pendleton wool and matching hand-knit sweaters and caps. The Boyntons were civilized in ways I had never seen. They did crossword puzzles in ink, drank sherry after church on Sunday, and shared names with their ancestors who'd come over on the *Mayflower*. At dinner, they discussed ideas.

When they finished a game of Boggle or Parcheesi, they returned the pieces neatly to their original boxes. They played Hearts and Spite and Malice with decks of cards that Larry's father had bought twenty-five years earlier. I had never seen such functional behavior. Our family room closet was stuffed with dismembered dolls, broken musical instruments, scattered Chinese checkers pieces, and an occasional empty soda can or half-eaten peanut butter sandwich. I'm pretty sure we didn't have a full deck of cards in the house, a metaphor lost on no one.

WHY CAN'T WE BE *more like that?* I asked when I went home at Christmas. Holmer laughed so hard, he spit out his nonalcoholic beer. He knew that I was the biggest culprit when it came to interrupting people at the dinner table, grabbing food off of someone else's plate, and making fart noises with my armpit, anything to keep the conversation light and silly.

Larry's mother made her own bread and jelly and decorated deviled eggs with slices of black olives and carrot shavings to look like penguins. The night I brought Larry home to Chicago to meet my family, my mother ordered takeout Chinese food. Larry knew all the rules of good etiquette from the many cotillion classes he took as a boy—which fork to use, how to wait to start eating until the hostess has taken her first bite, and so on. He sat patiently with his hand on his lap watching as we passed around the platter of egg rolls. The pile quickly shrank until just two were left by the time the plate made its way to Danny. Danny dumped both egg rolls on his plate and handed Larry the empty dish. Larry's mouth dropped open. He glared at me, but I had no sympathy for him.

If you're slow, you're skinny, I said, shrugging as I stuffed my egg roll in my mouth.

. . .

IF WE SPOKE ABOUT Nancy now, it was always with quick qualifiers: *She's in a better place, not suffering anymore, thank God.* But the shame and guilt of how she died lingered. I could see it on Patty's face most of all. In her senior year of nursing school, Patty was working forty hours or more as a home health aide to make money to pay her tuition. She was always an overachiever, working herself into a frazzle, not eating enough, getting very little sleep, sometimes not more than four hours a night.

In the winter of 1980, a year and a half after Nancy's death, Patty was assigned to her rotation in the psychiatric ward of a Milwaukee hospital. She shadowed doctors and nurses as they checked in on the patients who had either signed themselves in for emergency care or had been brought in by police. Many were suicidal. Some were dangerous to others. All were very sick. With all she had learned about mental illness from living with Nancy, Patty felt like this should have been her easiest rotation. Instead, it flattened her. She recalled the day Nancy died and how she stayed at her side, making her lunch, cleaning up her vomit, taking care to be certain that Nancy didn't fall asleep and risk slipping into a coma.

Why didn't I stay? Patty thought. *I never should have left her alone with Mom.*

She started having trouble sleeping. Her thoughts began to race.

It's just so sad, she told one of her supervisors. *I can't do it.* The woman asked her to explain. *I can't stop thinking of these patients and how much they are suffering,* Patty said. January in Milwaukee, with its gray skies, bitter cold, and howling winds, is challenging to even those with the stoutest spirit. The world looked like a very dark place to Patty. *Does this kind of sadness and dysfunction eventually catch up to us all?* she wondered. It sure felt like it to Patty. *I'm scared,* Patty told her supervisor. *I don't even know how to dig myself out of this hole of sadness, much less be able to help others do the same.*

Do you feel safe? the supervisor asked her.

I don't know, Patty said. At the woman's urging, Patty checked herself into the psych ward that afternoon. She slept, mostly, and after a day or two, she went back to school.

I didn't know any of this. None of us did. Patty told Holmer and our mother, who both encouraged her to do what she needed to do to feel better. But she did not confide in the rest of us.

Patty finished her rotation and graduated the following May. We sat in the auditorium bleachers and cheered as she received one of the nursing school's awards, unaware of its significance. It was the school's top honor in mental health nursing, and it came with a stipend that would go a long way to help Patty pay off her college loan. The woman who had encouraged Patty check into the psych ward months earlier nominated her for the award.

Never one to idle, Patty started her career as a nurse at Children's Hospital in Chicago the week after graduation. A few months later, she joined the Peace Corps, where she was assigned to a tiny village outside of Kinshasa in the Democratic Republic of the Congo, then known as Zaire.

"The more remote, the better," Patty said.

"I couldn't wait to get the hell out of Chicago and as far away from home as possible."

Several years later, I found a shoebox full of Patty's letters from the Peace Corps. She wrote about the stifling heat, the lack of running water and electricity, animals running through the streets, mud and insects everywhere. People were so poor, they slept five to a bed. And, yet, Patty had never known such joy.

"Everything is new to me—the food, the language, the sights, the sounds," Patty wrote. "I've never felt so alive!"

EVENTUALLY, WATERTOWN GREW ON me, and I came to see that I had a lot to learn from my fellow reporters. Many of them were just as skilled as anyone on the staff of *The New York Times* or *The Washington Post*. My assignments became more ambitious. I wrote a series of articles, no doubt informed by personal experience, about stressed-out high school kids and their poor mental health. But John Johnson was right. The city girl in me yearned for more action than a town that size could provide. I was spending most Saturday nights reading Truman Capote and John Irving books from the grandstands while Larry played ice hockey. Meanwhile, my college buddies were out whooping it up 750 miles west at the bars on Rush Street in Chicago. I started getting itchy.

My big break came that fall when I inadvertently broke one of the biggest stories in that area in decades: Abbie Hoffman, the Vietnam War–era counterculture hero, now wanted by the FBI, had been living on the lam, hiding out near Watertown for years under the name Barry Freed. We got the tip the day after Labor Day 1980. With a combination of sharp investigative techniques, dogged reporting, and dumb luck (mostly dumb luck), we nailed the story for our afternoon deadline and scooped the world.

The story had my byline on it, but it really was a team effort. Apparently, even Hoffman was impressed with our pluck and hustle. After deadline, I walked home to treat myself to a peanut butter and jelly sandwich, and when I returned to the newsroom there was yet another WHILE YOU WERE OUT message waiting for me at my desk. This one was from Hoffman, calling from New York City, in police custody. His three-word message:

"Nice work, kid."

The scoop yielded me a byline in *Newsweek* and a job offer covering cops for *The Cincinnati Post*.

I was sad to leave Larry but believed that if the romance was meant to be, we would find a way to keep it going long distance. His dad thought so, too.

"You leave behind a lot of friends and relatives who love you and count on you to stay in touch," his father wrote.

I left Watertown in January 1981, on the very day that the Iranian hostages were released as Ronald Reagan was being sworn in as the fortieth president of the United States. My mother, now fully sober for more than a year, met me at the Buffalo airport and helped drive me down to Cincinnati to get settled into my new apartment, conveniently located in the same building as Jane, one of my best friends from college. No janky transmissions this time. I unpacked my philodendron and fern and made sure the refrigerator was full.

LARRY MET ME AT the Albany County airport the night before Thanksgiving 1981 and, just as planned, handed me the black velvet box. During our Cape Cod vacation the month before, I told him it was time to fish or cut bait. *If this romance is to continue, we are getting married.* Larry agreed.

No dating service algorithm would ever put the two of us together—a flibbertigibbet Irish Catholic midwesterner and a taciturn WASP atheist from the East Coast. *Well, they're a nice couple, but I hear she's ROMAN Catholic!* I could hear Larry's grandmother declare from the other end of the dining room table one night. But the heart wants what it wants. We would find a way to make it work. After the trauma of Nancy's suicide and the years of fallout, I craved the stability that I knew Larry could offer me.

At twenty-four and still smitten by earthly treasures, I couldn't wait to see what kind of diamond ring he had picked out for me. Square-cut? A platinum setting just like the one Grandma had bought for my mother? Or gold, as I preferred? My hands trembled as I pawed the box open. To my horror, there was not a bright, shining diamond nestled within the velvet lining but an aluminum pull-tab to a beer can. I shot Larry a nasty glare.

If that doesn't fit, try this, he said, fishing out a thin gold band with a 0.20-carat diamond chip anchored in the middle. Typical Larry Boynton, grounding me to reality. After all, I was marrying a daily newspaper reporter, not an investment banker. I threw my arms around him and slid the ring on my finger, knowing he would never let me take myself too seriously or get lost, literally or figuratively.

Larry's father hooted when we walked in the door to announce the news. My new tribe welcomed me with unmitigated enthusiasm. Our wedding was set for late September.

Back at home, my mother sprang into action, lining up a venue for the reception, booking a band, making one list after another. At last, she found a way to pay back all her friends for the countless weddings she and Holmer attended. There would be parties and showers and gift registries. Place settings of silver and china, crystal goblets, and candlesticks. A honeymoon in Bermuda. We were giddy.

No one knew then what was about to hit us or how painful and humiliating the next year would turn out to be.

9

Love and a Hate Crime

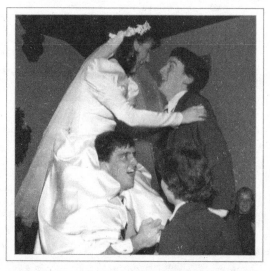

*The Chicken Fight: Me on Billy's shoulders, Danny, and
Chris Peters, our best man. Michigan Shores Club, Wilmette,
Illinois, 1982. (Courtesy of John Howell of John Howell
Studios, Winnetka, Illinois.)*

Danny was six years younger than I, so I looked at him with more maternal affection than as a typical sibling rival. We were too far apart in age to bicker. I always felt a little sorry for him, living in Billy's shadow. Everything seemed to come so easily for Billy. But Danny, two years younger to the day, was always a little bit behind, not quite as tall or dashing or skilled on the field of play. Danny was also elected vice president of his class at New Trier East High School and he played baseball but, comparatively, he was the underdog who could use a little cheering section.

I got a kick out of his quirky sense of humor, which usually came at his own expense. *I'm just a skinny man living in a fat man's world,* Danny used to say. My friends found him charming, too.

He came to visit me at DePauw for Little Sibling weekend a few months after Nancy died and stayed at the Delt fraternity house with some of my friends. Unbeknownst to me, Danny got on the loudspeaker there and invited all the brothers to brunch at my sorority house, not one bit concerned that I would be on the hook for the bill. I looked out the window that Sunday morning and saw Danny marching along like the Pied Piper with a trail of hungry Delts streaming toward the front door.

Danny started a lawn business when he was in high school, naming it YardBirds, an homage to Eric Clapton, his favorite guitarist. He had shirts made with the company logo, a wren pushing a lawn mower, and hired several of his friends. Even Billy did a little work for him, though Danny eventually fired him, claiming he took too long of a lunch break. By his senior year, Danny had built an operation of dozens of customers and had made enough money to buy an old red truck. He left for the University of Iowa that fall with plans of keeping the business running when he returned for holidays and summer break.

Danny looked frightened when he came into my bedroom one day just after Christmas that year. He closed the door. Danny sat on the edge of my bed and pulled out a story from the weekly community newspaper about a sixty-three-year-old man who owned Weiss Tire, a nearby tire store and truck repair shop. The story said someone was harassing the man by signing him up for magazine subscriptions made out in the names of Nazi war criminals like Heinrich Himmler and Josef Mengele. The man, obviously, was distraught. He was Jewish, and several of his family members had been killed by the Nazis in the Holocaust.

How awful, I said.

Danny stared at me for my reaction and said, *We did that.*

I could tell he was scared. He knew this "prank," as he called it, had gone too far, and he was groping for a way out. He described how he had been screwed over by the man, who, in Danny's opinion, charged him too much—$400 to fix his truck's brakes. When Danny had no luck getting the man to lower the bill, he and two of his high school friends, both of whom now also went to the University of Iowa, launched this secret campaign to get revenge.

This is really serious, I told Danny. I was shocked that he could have come up with something so vicious.

His confession to me seemed like a plea for help—he was trying to figure out what he should do next.

You need to get ahead of this, I told him. *Go to the police station and let them know what you did. Tell them you are sorry and put an end to it before it gets even more out of hand. You're going to get caught.*

But Danny ignored my advice.

I was working on a story in the *Cincinnati Post* newsroom on a Saturday a few weeks later when a dispatch came over the wires with the headline: THREE ARRESTED IN NAZI HATE MAILINGS. There was Danny's high school senior class photo alongside his two friends. The story was displayed on the front page of the *Chicago Tribune,* January 11, 1982—which also happened to be Danny's nineteenth birthday.

The police, with the help of postal service inspectors and other federal agencies, had been able to trace the subscription orders back to Danny and his friends. In addition to the magazine subscriptions, they'd sent Mailgrams to dozens of the man's customers, impersonating him and saying he would not service them because they were "Semitic." They also took out ads in Chicago-area newspapers under the man's name, selling tires for ridiculously high prices. The whole campaign was as stupid as it was cruel.

I was mortified. It was hard to reconcile how Danny could be involved in something as sinister as this. Sure, all of us in our family were a little immature and tone-deaf when it came to our humor. But this was an orchestrated campaign of hate that had gone on for more than two months. Couldn't he understand how wrong this was, how painful this was for this man and his family?

Danny was arrested at home and taken into custody, where he was fingerprinted, photographed, and charged with felony theft and disorderly conduct, a misdemeanor. He and the two others pleaded not guilty at their arraignment and were each released on $2,000 bond. The Chicago media ate it up, and I understood exactly why.

This story had all the elements that I looked for in my own stories: outrage, a sympathetic victim, and entitled villains. Three handsome, privileged young men who had graduated from one of the most prominent high schools in the country, now in their freshman year of college, had been charged with a crime so mean-spirited that it was hard to discuss without feeling disgusted. They cast Danny and his accomplices as modern-day Leopolds and Loebs.

As much as I wanted to, I couldn't rip this story out and hide it in my socks and underwear drawer the way I had done with the story about Nancy and the train. Danny's case was covered by every medium—TV and radio and newspapers all over the country, including *The New York Times* and, to my particular humiliation, my employer, *The Cincinnati Post*. Reporters started calling and showing up at the house on Greenwood Avenue. They interviewed the neighbors, wondering what kind of people my parents were that they could raise someone as despicable as Danny. It would have been easier for Frazier Thomas, our neighbor, the children's television show host, to say nothing, considering the risk of offending his viewers. But he generously told the reporters that my parents were good people and fine next-door neighbors.

Whatever you do, don't talk to the reporters, I told Danny. I knew that anything he said could get twisted. Reporters were looking for any way to feed into the narrative about privileged North Shore teens acting cruelly. But it was too late. Any hopes we had that this would go away easily were dashed once Danny opened his mouth. Once again, he ignored my advice. He told a reporter for the *Chicago Tribune* that he was "the real victim" because "I'm being blamed for what I didn't do." He said the only reason his name had been mentioned was that he knew the two culprits. He was trying to lay it all on his two friends. As I feared, the reporter wasted no time turning that into another big headline. I probably would have done the same thing. Now, in the eyes of the reader, Danny wasn't just cruel, he was conniving and dishonest, a weasel who was trying to blame others for the hateful things he had done.

My parents' home phone started to ring nonstop.

I hope your son goes to prison and gets raped, one woman said.

He should be shot, said another.

My family had just sat down for dinner one night when a man burst through the front door, screaming that Danny deserved to die. *You all do,* the man said, glaring at my mother. *Shame on you.* The Wilmette police started guarding the house.

As the media fascination intensified, the case became about more than just Danny and his friends and their hateful actions. Larger forces were at work, greater consequences at stake. Just a few years earlier, a Nazi group announced plans to demonstrate in Skokie, the town next to Wilmette, where the man who owned the tire shop lived. The group chose that venue because of its high concentration of Holocaust survivors, then one in every six of the village's Jewish citizens. Skokie officials ignored the group's request for a permit, then filed an injunction to prevent the parade. The American Civil Liberties Union challenged the injunction, claiming it violated the group's First Amendment right to free speech.

The case eventually made its way to the U.S. Supreme Court. The justices refused to overturn the lower-court ruling that the Nazis had a constitutional right to march.

Members of the Anti-Defamation League were now lobbying to strengthen the national hate crime statute. They met with the judge, urging him to keep in mind how important Danny's case was. The Skokie decision had been a great blow. *Anti-Semitism like this cannot be tolerated,* they said. *Anything less than full prosecution leaves a crack in the door for hatred to spread everywhere. We need to make a statement with this case while all eyes are on it.*

Danny's trial was set for June, three months before Larry and I were scheduled to get married. Danny went back to school in Iowa to begin his second semester, hoping the infamy would not catch up to him there and that he would somehow be able to concentrate on his studies. But he was wrong. He lay in bed thinking of the trouble he was now in, growing increasingly agitated and depressed, scared of what might happen.

Holmer suggested that Danny talk to a priest. *Turn it over to God,* Holmer said. That had worked for him when he quit drinking. He was hoping an Act of Contrition would do the same for Danny. Danny found a parish near campus. The man heard Danny's story and encouraged him to stay the night. *You look pretty upset, Dan,* the priest told him. *We'll take good care of you here.* He settled Danny into a room at the rectory. A few hours later, Danny woke up to find the priest standing over his bed, reaching under the covers to fondle him. *I ran out of there as fast as I could,* Danny later told me.

None of us could escape the notoriety of Danny's case. I was driving home to Chicago for the weekend to register for wedding gifts when a story came on the radio giving tips to parents on how to not raise children like Danny and his friends.

Patty, now a registered nurse on her way to the Peace Corps, was so embarrassed at the nearly daily dose of media coverage labeling Danny as a "hate-spewing bigot" that she took off her name tag at work. The attention was especially hard on Molly, who was a senior at New Trier and had to go to school every day enduring the stares and whispers of her classmates as the story unfolded on the nightly news and in daily newspapers.

All I wanted to think about was my wedding planning and whether to go with the dusty-rose bath towels or mint green, or both. It seemed surreal to be focusing on wedding flower arrangements and which readings about love to pick for the ceremony when my little brother was on trial for such a hateful crime.

Danny's legal troubles had renewed Holmer's interest in the law. Over the past several months, he had been studying to take the Illinois bar exam. Though Holmer had graduated from law school nearly thirty years earlier, he never established a legal practice. He was too busy chasing big advertising deals, until his career started to fizzle. If he wanted to practice now, he would have to pass the Illinois bar exam. We made plenty of jokes about Holmer having trouble passing any bar—particularly those that served alcohol—but we admired the grit of our sixty-year-old father studying alongside some of our friends who were just getting out of law school.

Larry and I were in Wilmette one April weekend, a few months before our wedding, to meet with Father Hartmann, the St. Francis priest who would be presiding at our ceremony. Unlike my Grandpa Matt, who had been henpecked into converting, Larry had no interest in becoming Catholic. The eight years he spent singing in his Episcopal church's men's and boys' choir were more than enough organized religion for him. His father used to say that Larry was "allergic to stained glass." But Larry knew how important my faith was to me, even if he wanted no part of it. Nothing could sway him, not even when one of Holmer's cousins gave him a Catholic version of the Bible the size of some coffee tables. But in order to have our union blessed by the Catholic Church, Larry and I would need to participate in marriage training, known as Pre-Cana, which Larry kept referring to as "Pre-Carnal."

Let me get this straight, Larry said. *A guy who has never been married gets to tell us if we can get married or not?*

Yep, I said. *Pretty much. Welcome to the Catholic Church. Basically, you have to promise to "accept children lovingly from God" and then agree to raise them in the church.*

Hmmmmm, Larry growled.

Larry is a tough customer. He wasn't going to agree to something if he didn't want to. I worried that he might push back so hard that the priest would refuse to perform the ceremony. The three of us talked for a while, and then Father Hartmann had me leave the room. *Oh, shit,* I thought and gave Larry a long pleading glance.

How'd it go in there? I nervously asked Larry as we drove back to the house on Greenwood.

I said what I needed to say, said Larry, offering no more details. As far as I knew, the wedding was still on, but I couldn't be 100 percent certain.

Early that evening, Mary Kay called home with a big announcement.

She and her boyfriend Tom had eloped at city hall with Jeanie Beanski, their miniature poodle, as the attendant.

My mother's face fell when she heard the news, not because she didn't approve of Tom but because she had missed out on a chance to plan another wedding. We were delighted for them, but confused. How many times had we heard Mary Kay say that she was never going to get married?

When Holmer walked in the door the next day, wondering what might be new, my mother greeted him with the one-two punch: *Well, you flunked the bar exam, and Mary Kay got married.* He stood there for a long time, blinking.

If my parents' feelings were hurt that their oldest child had left them and all of us out of their wedding plans, they didn't say so. My mother shifted gears to hosting a dinner for Mary Kay and Tom. Holmer enrolled in another law school refresher course with plans to retake the bar exam the next time it was offered.

I stayed busy covering the stories on my beat—murder trials, corporate theft, and the Hamilton County, Ohio, prosecution of *Hustler* magazine publisher Larry Flynt on charges of obscenity. But the court case that captured most of my attention was three hundred miles north at the Cook County courthouse, where my little brother Danny was about to go on trial.

The picture for Danny was darkening by the day. His two codefendants, clearly stung by Danny's remarks to the *Tribune* reporter, agreed to testify against him in exchange for plea deals. The rats were chewing on each other. Prosecutors had reduced the charges to misdemeanors, hoping to goose a plea out of Danny, too. But he was hell-bent on fighting, and my parents, against their friends' and families' best advice, reluctantly went along.

Danny was so ashamed of his role in this that he had convinced himself he was innocent. He would rather mount a ridiculous defense than admit to his role in these crimes. My parents felt they had to let Danny have his day in court. We all knew Danny was guilty. But, just as they had ignored the doctor's counsel and let Nancy go off to Boulder, Colorado, to school, they wanted to give Danny the benefit of the doubt. The results were equally disastrous.

The bench trial began on June 28, 1982, and lasted three days. It drew hundreds of spectators, including A. Abbot Rosen, the Midwest director of the Anti-Defamation League, who met with reporters after each session to discuss the case. Tens of thousands of people followed it on the news each day.

All the attention had shifted to Danny, since the other two had agreed to take plea deals. Danny had taken a terrible situation and made it substantially worse by clinging to his false narrative that he was innocent. The prosecution had built a strong case. They had lined up one of Danny's old customers who had squabbled with Danny over a bill for eleven dollars. She said Danny told her he "didn't like working for Jews."

But the real blow to Danny's case came the next day when one of his codefendants took the stand and testified that he had seen Danny dressed up like Hitler for Halloween, a claim Danny denied. In headlines, Danny was now known as the "Nazi prankster." Even Danny's own lawyer didn't have a comeback for that. "If there's a crime charging an 18- or 19-year-old boy with being an anti-Semite, then the state has a good case."

No one except Danny was surprised when the judge found him guilty.

"I wish I could send you to Dachau," the judge told Danny. "But I can't." He sentenced Danny to four weekends in the Cook County jail.

A dozen or more reporters followed the tire shop owner into the hallway after the verdict was announced, hoping to get his reaction.

"I'm very happy with the verdict," the man said. "I can't tell you what it was like to go through this."

Rosen hailed the verdict as a "signal to the bigots out there that this sort of conduct is impermissible." I agreed with every word he said, even as my heart was breaking for my stupid brother.

The next morning, Danny and Holmer were pictured on the *Tribune*'s front page, scowling as they exited the courthouse. My mother trailed behind looking lost and ashamed.

At least we'll get this behind us now, I thought. *Let's accept the verdict, do your jail time, and move on.* But no. Now Danny wanted to appeal.

No way, I thought. As far as I was concerned, this would just delay the inevitable for another several months. This was agony for us all, especially that poor man who owned the tire store. Once again, my parents went along with it.

We couldn't endlessly dwell on Danny's trial. Larry's and my wedding was less than three months away, a Mass at St. Francis Xavier, followed by a sit-down dinner for 285 guests at the Michigan Shores Club, sponsored by my dad's cousin Joe, since we, of course, were no longer members. I wasn't about to let this humiliating spectacle ruin our big day. I'm sure people whispered behind our backs about this most unfortunate family. First, a dead sister; now, a disgraced brother. But we kept our game faces glowing.

Good to see you all here tonight, Holmer said in the opening remarks of his father-of-the-bride toast. *I know you've been seeing a lot of us lately.* People laughed nervously. *Oh, God,* I thought, *don't go there.*

Then he introduced my mother as his "sex partner of the last thirty-one years." I gazed out at my in-laws, wondering how they were taking all of this. A few minutes later, the music started. We rushed to the dance floor.

Suddenly, I was hoisted onto Billy's shoulders, doing a chicken fight with Danny, who had climbed on top of the best man. The photographer snapped a photo of Danny's eyes and mine locked in delight, blissfully tuning out anything else going on around us. Pure, unmitigated joy. On that night—in that moment, anyway—all I could think of was how grateful I was to be marrying a man whom I loved, who also loved me. He would provide me with some stability, even with all this crazy family baggage.

I stared into Danny's eyes, thinking, *Let this be the end of your troubles, too. Put this awful chapter behind you. Move forward, make something of your life. Find someone who will love you for who you are—crazy and flawed, with an irresistible zest for life. You've got so much going for you; you're young and handsome and funny. You can recover from this.*

But the rejoicing was only temporary, a short respite from the mess that Danny created.

AS PREDICTED, THE APPELLATE court affirmed Danny's conviction the following spring. He would have to go to jail after all, during the day for four consecutive weekends. I drove in from Cincinnati that first weekend to show him support. I hated what Danny did, but he was my brother, and I wanted to do what I could to help him get through this terrible chapter of his life. He came home at dinnertime, looking even paler than normal, his eyes blinking. This tic of his started just after Nancy died and grew worse each year. Danny refused dinner. He went right to the family room, lay on the floor next to the heater, and curled up in a fetal position.

A month later, when his sentence had been served, Danny came to Cincinnati at my urging to stay with Larry and me for some rest and to get away from Chicago. He slept a lot those first few days. When he was awake, he looked like a whipped dog, sometimes whimpering and shaking. That Saturday, I convinced him to come with me to five o'clock Mass at the cathedral downtown. We would go out after that for some ribs and cold beer. Mass always made me feel better, helped to calm me, and I was hoping it would do the same for Danny. I like the consistency that the rituals offer, how they remain the same even as our lives veer in and out of chaos. I find strength and courage in the words of the Gospel that remind us that we are all flawed and we all suffer. We cope with our pain by loving one another as we want to be loved. *Come with me,* I said. *It'll be good for you.* Reluctantly, Danny agreed.

As I'd hoped, Danny began to relax at Mass. We hugged at the sign of peace. *Maybe he'll bounce back in time,* I thought.

Then we saw them.

The bank of TV cameras drew closer as we headed out the door after Communion.

Oh, shit, I said. *They've followed us.*

A thick row of camera operators and reporters with their notebooks at the ready stood in a scrum lining the steps. Many were the very same reporters who had covered Danny's trial and chased him and Holmer down the block, shouting, *Do you think the Holocaust was fake? Why did you do it, Dan?*

Danny started to shake. I thought he might faint.

Keep moving, I told him as I grabbed his arm.

But they weren't there to interview us. The reporters hadn't even seen us. They had come from Chicago to interview Joseph Bernardin, the archbishop of Cincinnati, the man who had just said Mass that day. As we later learned, the pope had just named Bernardin as archbishop of Chicago, the largest archdiocese in the nation. He would soon be installed as a cardinal.

From the look of terror in Danny's eyes as we exited the church, I could see then that he would never shake off the shame of his cruel hoax, not that day, not ever.

10

Arrivals and Departures

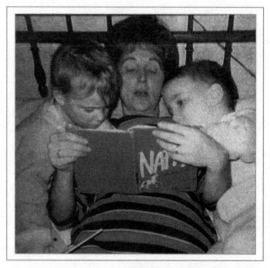

*Bedtime. My mother with Molly and Danny, a.k.a. the
Diapered Duo. Wilmette, Illinois, 1965.*

By August 1986, I was eight months pregnant with our first child and more than a little nervous about giving birth. Larry and I had moved to Milwaukee, knowing we wanted to start a family someday and live closer to his parents or mine. Milwaukee was as close as we got. I was covering the courts and writing about legal issues for *The Milwaukee Journal.* As my due date drew near, I began to panic. *How the hell is a baby's head supposed to get out of my body?* I asked my mother.

Beats me, she said. *God must be a man or he would have figured out an easier way.*

This was a cute answer, but, like those she gave to so many of the questions I had asked over the years about childbirth and caring for newborns, not a very satisfying one.

My mother came up to Milwaukee to help us when Charley was born, and then again, seventeen months later, when Molly, our daughter, arrived. In many ways, those were magical days. I had my mother's undivided attention for a full week. She was here for me, stone-cold sober and eager to help fold laundry, make dinner, and coo at these wonderful, squiggly new creatures. But I had so many questions, almost none that she could answer.

What do I do if he won't latch on?

My mother shrugged.

Should I give him a bath before his nap or after?

She shrugged again.

Is this colic?

Here a shrug. There a shrug. Everywhere a shrug shrug.

What do you mean you don't know? I asked her. *You had eight of these things.*

I don't remember, she said.

At first, I thought she was just trying to be polite, deferential, not overbearing, to let me discover the joy of motherhood on my own time, at my own pace. But I wanted direction, some practical advice that I could use to help me care for my newborns.

After about the tenth time she told me I would figure it out, I finally realized that she wasn't being coy. She genuinely did not remember. All those kids. All that laundry. All those feedings in the middle of the night. We were a blur to her now. She had been so overwhelmed by all of us—or by the gin and Valium—that the memories of those delicate, precious days had disappeared.

If I had any doubt about this, they were erased when Larry's mother, Barbara, came to stay with us the next week. Barbara had lots of useful tips for me:

- Put a diaper pin on the side where the baby last nursed so you will know to start with the other side next.

- Baths make babies sleepy.
- Stay away from broccoli when you are nursing. (It gives the baby gas.)

Larry was the first of Barbara's three children. So, understandably, she was an especially diligent, attentive mother with him. She kept meticulous notes, recording every feeding, poop, pee, smile, and precise length of his naps. My mother had no time or temperament for such things—especially with me. I had no baby book, not even the slightest record of my first years. I didn't see a baby picture of myself until my mother found a few negatives while she was cleaning out a drawer when I was in college.

I don't doubt that my mother loved each of us and, even if she had a choice, she would still have kids. Maybe not eight. Maybe not even four. In more ways than I can count, my mother was caring and loving. She just couldn't tell you how to get a baby on a sleep schedule if you put a gun to her head. I was hoping my mother could calm me down about my anxiety over giving birth. But, I learned, she had no idea whatsoever about how to manage the throes of labor. I found that to be so odd until I learned the disturbing reason why.

In her day, women in labor were put into a drug-induced trance, a procedure known as *twilight sleep*. With the help of a drug called *scopolamine* (also known as the date rape drug, "the Devil's Breath"), women felt the pain of giving birth; they just couldn't remember it. If she was too loopy to push, my mother would lie on the table like a stunned cow before the slaughter while the doctor grabbed a pair of forceps and yanked out one or the other of us. Eventually, she would "come to," to find yet another frantic, cone-headed newborn in her arms and stitches in her perineum, clueless of how either came about.

Even considering this overly medicalized way my mother gave birth to each of us, her amnesia about caring for babies, newborns in particular, was abnormal. She was held back from us by a gauze of her lifelong anxiety and ensuing postpartum depression. My mother could see us. She just could not get to us, completely. Each birth—blessed event though it was billed to be—was also a form of trauma for her, one that deprived her of memory and now my siblings and me the benefit of her expertise.

Nor could she be much help in advising me on how to handle a temperamental toddler. Determined not to repeat our family dynamic of "slap first, ask questions later" when some kid started to howl, I enrolled in a class at the nearby Jewish Community Center titled "How to Talk So Kids Will Listen & Listen So Kids Will Talk," based on the book of the same name by Adele Faber and Elaine Mazlish. I taped the advice on the inside of the cabinets in the kitchen and bathrooms for ready reference. *Huh,* my mother said as she opened our kitchen cabinet one morning and read a section on how to de-escalate a tantrum. *Whadaya know about that!*

As overwhelmed as she appeared to be about raising all of us, my mother relished her role as grandmother. She seemed tailor-made for the job, knitting my children and Mary Kay's little sweaters, making them Easter baskets, spoiling them with Teenage Mutant Ninja Turtles or stuffed rabbits. Now that she had quit drinking, she was clear-eyed and focused, relaxed and confident. She would bundle up those babies and stroll them around the block, even on the coldest winter day.

Fresh air, she would say, yanking the stroller through the door. *Shakes the stink off of them.*

Grateful for this new connection with her, I would go down to Wilmette any chance I could get. I relished the one-on-one time with my mother that I was never able to have as a kid. I wanted to be around her as often as I could, to make up for lost time.

I found her charming and brilliant and hilarious. Unwittingly, we started dressing alike in denim jumpers with plaid turtlenecks, complete with shoulder pads, and leather flats, the classic '80s suburban mom getup. I even went to her hairdresser. We had twin perms! We bought the same dining room set and the same Waverly wallpaper for our bathrooms. *Oh my God,* my old pal Mary Claire said when we bumped into her coming out of the dry cleaners one day. *You're turning into your mother.* For the first time in a long time, maybe ever, I considered that a compliment.

Once the source of my frustration and bitter disappointment—and, if I am being brutally honest, disdain—my mother was fast becoming my role model, someone I looked to for strength. Quitting drinking had made her strong in ways I never imagined that she could be. It gave her a sense of accomplishment that we all admired. She looked younger and healthier. She took tennis lessons and ballet. She and Holmer joined a cooking club. On the weeks when she was assigned to run her home group's AA meeting, my attention-averse mother would dutifully type up her testimonials and muster the courage to admit to how powerless she had been over booze. *I'm so thankful to finally be sober,* she would often say.

Her enthusiasm for these meetings ran so hot that it occasionally got her in trouble.

Say, I saw [fill in the blank], she'd say to one of us, recalling one of our grade school teachers or the coach of one of our old sports teams.

Oh yeah? we would answer. *Where?*

Then my mother's face would freeze.

Can't say, she'd quickly answer.

And then we knew. She had taken the A out of AA.

A few months after Charley was born, with my mother's help, I discovered the power of telling my story, too. Not about a battle with the bottle but, fittingly, a fussy baby. It was a ghost story.

Charley and I were visiting my parents one January weekend, bunking in my childhood bedroom, home of the infamous Tiger Pit. Charley, who was about five months old, had spiked a fever from a case of roseola. By 2 a.m., the little guy was so miserable, he could not sleep. I rocked him in my lap to get him to quiet down so he wouldn't wake the whole house. I reached for something to read to him, but the only book within my grasp was my old high school yearbook. As I began leafing through the pages, I noticed something I had never seen.

Someone had gone through and put devil's horns on my picture and blackened out a tooth, then wrote notes in the margins, pretending to be a friend of mine. *Let's get drunk this weekend on (picture of a beer mug).* I recognized the handwriting immediately—and also the snark. This could only be the sinister handiwork of one person! How is it that I had never seen the notes Nancy had written?

With every page I turned, more goofy drawings. Nancy, dead for more than eight years by then, was still finding ways to mess with me. This was the spirit of the funny Nancy, front-porch-sing-along sister, not the swallow-a-bottle-of-pills-and-lock-yourself-in-the-bathroom variety. As I sat in my old bedroom in the predawn darkness, I was overwhelmed thinking about how much I missed her then and how I wished she could have met my baby boy.

Back in Milwaukee a few days later, I fired off an essay about coming across those drawings and how it felt like Nancy had come back from the grave all these years later to share in a little fun. I was full of maternal hormones and ached for Charley to know about her—the good and the bad, how she dyed my hair when I was too young for such a thing, how she used to stick her wads of chewed gum under the kitchen table and on the headboard of her four-poster bed, how she chased me with a knife when I tried to steal her sweaters, how she strummed the guitar off-key, how she could play "Für Elise" by third grade. She was beautiful and horrible and hilarious and vicious as hell. She was my sister, and I loved her. I had been relieved when she died, but now, I missed her terribly.

I had not let myself remember Nancy like that because I was too ashamed of the way she died. Trauma does that to you. It steals your memory. I either couldn't or didn't let myself remember her or talk about her. But here she was. Dead or not, Nancy had showed up to goof around with me a bit.

I shared my essay with the editor of the newspaper's Sunday magazine. He loved it. Confessionals about suicide were not common in daily newspapers in 1987. Most newspapers had a policy of not mentioning suicide in obituaries, for fear they would scandalize the families. My editor commissioned an artist to draw a portrait of Nancy and put my essay on the cover of the magazine. The portrait featured Nancy from her Janis Joplin phase, with bright orange flames framing her face.

Holmer was livid when the piece came out, though I had told him that

I was writing it. He was angry that I had included the fact that Nancy had killed herself.

You don't need to tell anyone about that, he said. *That's none of their business.*

My mother jumped right in.

Yes, she does, Bill, my mother said. *That's how she makes sense of it.*

My mother had been to hundreds of AA meetings by then. She had heard just about everything people can do to humiliate themselves under the power of alcohol and drugs—the lies and cover-ups, the crazy places they hid their liquor bottles, the cockamamie excuses they gave. Some of the stories were hilarious. All of them were heartbreaking.

Meg needs to tell this story, Bill, my mother said. Her tone was as sure and strong as I had ever heard it. Eventually, Holmer came to see the merits of it.

I was terrified to go into the newsroom the day after the story ran, afraid everyone would be staring at me. *Her sister jumped in front of a train!* The elevator doors opened, and I slinked to my desk, trying to avoid eye contact. *That was some story,* said the medical reporter whose desk was next to mine. *Good for you.* Colleagues I had never really talked to before stopped by my desk to hug me and to thank me for sharing my story. A quiet man on the copy desk told me his son died like that, too.

Later that day, my phone rang. The director of the Big Brothers Big Sisters of Milwaukee was calling to congratulate me on my story, but, he said, there was one thing that he couldn't figure out. A few years earlier, I volunteered to be a mentor to a girl whose parents had divorced and who needed a little extra attention. I would spend Saturdays or Sundays with her, baking cookies, going on walks or to the movies. I took her to the newsroom softball games and carved pumpkins with her at Halloween. When I applied for the role, I filled out a long questionnaire about my background, including the names and occupations of all my family members.

I thought you told me your sister Nancy was a music teacher, he said. Long pause.

My throat closed. My eyes started to sting.

I had told him that. When I filled out the application, I had been too embarrassed to tell him the real story, afraid he would think that there might be something wrong with me, too. Maybe mental illness ran in the family. People are always assuming that having a mental illness makes someone dangerous, though that is rarely true. Maybe he thought I would hurt someone. So, I lied and said Nancy taught music.

Oh, yeah, I said. *Sorry about that.*

After I hung up, I went and hid in a stall in the ladies' room so no one could hear me crying. Poor Nancy. She wasn't a music teacher. She wanted to be, but she was too sick to finish school. That's the real story. She was sick and nothing she tried or we tried could make her better. And when she couldn't stand it any longer, she jumped in front of a train because she would rather get crushed to death than live one more second in that much pain. I'm glad I could set the record straight. Nancy deserved to be remembered for the way she really was, not for how we wanted her to be.

BY 1990, THE HOUSE on Greenwood Avenue had become too much for Holmer and my mother to afford and maintain. Jake, who was working in the plumbing department of a nearby hardware store, was still living at home, but everyone else had scattered. My parents didn't need that beast of a house with its seven bedrooms and four bathrooms anymore. Besides, housing prices were skyrocketing, and, with Holmer's shaky employment record, they could use the cash.

Aside from houses on the Lake Michigan shore, our little section of east Wilmette was the most desirable of our suburb, and the price tags for the houses reflected that. Leaving the house we grew up in felt like another death in a way. It was hard to let go. Like each of us, that house had seen a lot of sorrow, but somehow still managed to be a source of great joy and welcoming to all. No one was too eccentric, drunk, or disheveled to be denied a place at the Kissinger dinner table. Our house was the spot all our friends gathered on summer nights and on weekends. We never locked the door. People knew to just come inside and not to bother ringing the door bell.

My parents pretended to be excited about the move, and we hosted a blowout Goodbye House party. Each kid could invite ten friends. We carved our initials into a beam in the basement where the crickets chirped each night.

My parents bought a three-bedroom town house about a mile away that Holmer irreverently called "the projects." When we were cleaning out the house on Greenwood, I found a rotten egg in a Tampax box that my mother had hidden one Easter many years earlier. Mary Kay found another one in the hutch in the dining room. *Imagine*, I thought, *how many other treasures—and secrets—have been buried, never to be found, in this place over the last quarter of a century.*

Our new place will feel like home in no time, my mother promised. But it never did, especially after the bruises on her legs started showing up— one after another, after another.

SHE THOUGHT AT FIRST that the spots on her leg were from bumping into the new dishwasher. *I'm just not used to the new kitchen*, my mother said. When she started spiking fevers, she knew it was time for her to see a doctor.

I was making macaroni and cheese for my kids when she and Holmer called me with news of what the tests revealed. The conversation went like this:

Holmer: Hey, Grunt [his most recent nickname for me]. Let's say you're at a party and someone says, "Everyone here whose mother does not have cancer, raise your hand." Do you raise your hand?

Me: [heart pounding] Should I?

Holmer: Not so fast.

My mother had been diagnosed with non-Hodgkin lymphoma, small cell. The doctors said her chances for survival depended on how well she responded to the chemotherapy. I tossed and turned all that night and went down to see her the next day. By the next week, the week before Christmas, my mother was still in the hospital, very weak. For months, Larry and I had planned to take our kids on the train to Albany to spend Christmas with his family. His dad, Nat, a train buff, was so excited that he drew us a little diagram of how the four of us could fit in the tiny roomette we had reserved.

No way am I leaving my mother, I told Larry. *This could very well be her last Christmas.*

But my father-in-law insisted that we come.

You're not going to change anything by being away, he said. I was shocked by his callousness.

I loved my father-in-law. Nat Boynton was a warm, smart, principled, gregarious guy and a great storyteller. Like me, he had started his newspaper career at the *Watertown Daily Times.* He went on to become the sports editor in Geneva, New York, before joining the Associated Press covering the New York legislature. Like me, he was a baseball nut. We spent hours talking by the fire, sipping sherry or draining bottles of cold beer, discussing classic newspaper ledes, our favorite "URs" (his cheeky list of "unnecessary redundancies," like "free gift"), or the questionable merit of the designated hitter rule.

Nat was a brilliant writer and easily could have climbed the corporate ladder at General Electric, a pantheon for wordsmiths that once included the future great novelist Kurt Vonnegut. Nat's heart was in journalism, but he figured, reasonably, that he could not provide well enough for a family on a reporter's salary. He wrote speeches for the company executives and put together corporate slide presentations. Nat turned down many offers of promotion, not wanting to uproot his family and move to New York City. By his calculations, a well-balanced life was more valuable than any executive privileges. He'd rather spend weekends skiing and fishing with his children and friends than working overtime to impress some boss many years his junior.

I admired his priorities. We had even more in common, as it turned out. Not long before Larry and I got married, Nat had confided something to me that he'd never told his own children. They knew that Nat's mother, their grandmother, had died of a blood clot at the age of forty-nine, complications from a broken leg. Larry and his sisters were always told that their grandfather had died exactly a year later of a broken heart.

The more specific cause was a lot more disturbing. He had shot himself in the head, leaving Nat, nineteen, a sophomore at Princeton, and his two younger sisters orphaned in the height of the Great Depression.

I could not imagine how anyone could climb out of that hole, but here was Nat: successful, adored by his family, amused by his friends, admired by many, unafraid to stand up for what he saw as wrong, and, still, one of the most cheerful people I ever met.

How did you find the strength to keep going? I asked him. I knew from Nancy's death and, even more so, my mother's near suicide a few years earlier, how bitter that can make a person feel, so unimportant and abandoned.

I had a choice, Nat told me. *I could feel sorry for myself and wallow in pity or choose to be happy and do what I could to make that happen.*

Everything about Nat's life seemed to be an intentional act to overcome his family tragedies. The example he set had buoyed me dozens of times over the years. I looked at Nat as a role model in every way—the very picture of resilience. But his demand that we come that Christmas seemed selfish. My mother was dying.

As I was planning to cancel the trip, my mother started to rally. Her cheeks pinked up. Her appetite returned. The doctor said her blood work looked great. She was bouncing back.

Go, she said. *I'll be here when you get back.*

Larry and the kids and I boarded the train and took our spots in the roomette just as Nat had advised. We woke up on Christmas Eve morning to snow falling gently on the ground outside of Buffalo. It felt like a dream, like we were floating on the pages of *The Polar Express.* We sipped hot chocolate in the club car and sang Christmas carols. Nat was beaming when he met us later that day at the station in Rensselaer.

When I called home on Christmas night, Holmer sounded winded, distracted. After a few surface comments about Christmas, he delivered the blow. *Well, she's not home yet,* he said. *They're going to keep her in the hospital for a few more days. Um.* He paused. *She's been transferred to the psych ward.*

What?

Danny had been to visit her in the oncology ward earlier that night and said she seemed fine. But, after he left, a nurse discovered my mother lying in a pool of her own blood. She had tried to cut open her veins with some scissors she used for her knitting.

I felt like throwing up. How could she do this to us, again? Just like passing out in the attic or that morning in Elkhart, Indiana, when I found her drinking a martini, this seemed so weak and selfish. She was our mother. She was a freaking grandmother! She knew the toll Nancy's suicide had taken on us all—especially her. Did any of that matter to her? Did she pause to consider how shattered we would all be if she killed herself in the goddamn oncology ward?

We had spent weeks sitting by her bed, praying, decorating her room with a little Christmas tree, taping pictures of us and the grandkids on the walls. We hoped that would be incentive for her to fight the good fight. She was only sixty-four years old. So much to live for. We needed her.

We had implored the doctors and nurses to do their best to make our mother better, and now she was going to ruin it all by killing herself? I was so angry I could not see straight. I excused myself to my in-laws, went upstairs, and sobbed into my pillow. I never told them what had happened.

As I lay in bed, I thought about my own two kids, asleep in the next room. I couldn't imagine leaving them like that. How could my mother do this to us? Again. In my anguish that night, I could not see what I have now come to understand—that she was not acting rationally. She wasn't thinking of me or Holmer or my brothers and sisters, or any of the grandchildren. She couldn't think of anything but the pain she was in.

She was not trying to kill herself, she told Billy and Patty the next day. The prednisone they gave her to help fight the lymphoma had made her hallucinate. She was out of her mind, convinced that the pictures on the walls were dancing and that the doctors and nurses were all drunk. *There's a liquor store right across the street, you know,* she told Holmer. I wasn't sure I bought this explanation.

If she wasn't thinking clearly, why hadn't the doctors and nurses paid more attention to her? Steroids are known to increase the likelihood of suicide, especially for patients like my mother, with a history of depression and anxiety. They should have been watching her more carefully.

By the time Larry, the kids, and I returned from Albany a few days later, my mother was home from the hospital. Still shaken, I drove down to Chicago to see her the next day, trying not to stare at the gauze around her wrist. Of course, I never asked her about this suicide attempt, and she did not offer any explanation or apology or discuss it in any way. It was just another trauma to sweep away, unaddressed. Move right along.

In hindsight, I'm glad that Nat insisted that we spend Christmas with them that year. Less than two weeks after our visit, our kitchen phone rang. Larry's mother was calling with terrible news. Nat collapsed that morning at church. The paramedics rushed in to save him, but it was too late. His heart had stopped. Nat died at the hospital that afternoon. The other half of the grapefruit he had eaten that morning was still in the refrigerator when Larry and I flew out there the next day to be with his mother and sisters and baby nephew.

The following month, my mother went back to Lad & Lassie, the children's clothing store where she had been working for the past few years. Holmer started calling her "Lazarus," because, he said, just like the biblical character, she had come back from the dead.

Even Lazarus's staying power had his limits. By the next spring, my mother had battled back two more rounds of lymphoma. Each time the cancer returned, she rallied but grew weaker. Mouth sores, bruises, overwhelming fatigue. In between, she tried squeezing as much out of life while the getting was good. My parents traveled to New Orleans to watch Patty get her doctorate in epidemiology. She helped watch Mary Kay's two boys, Ryan and Connor, while Mary Kay was on bed rest, pregnant with her daughter, Devin. Holmer resorted to his usual gallows humor to cope with the tension of watching my mother battle a deadly disease. He told her how much he loved her Thanksgiving stuffing—made of pork sausage, celery, onions, and butter—and, now that she was feeling better, could she make a few extra batches and put them in the freezer just in case? The following August, she started spiking fevers again.

ARRIVALS OR DEPARTURES? MY mother never could figure out the overhead traffic signs at O'Hare International, Chicago's main airport. Upper level for departures, lower level for arrivals.

Well, I'm arriving at the airport, but he's departing, she would say as she drove to pick up Holmer on Fridays after his weekly business trips to New York.

Now, Labor Day weekend of 1992, I was arriving at the airport to fetch Patty from New Orleans and Molly from Utah so they could say goodbye to our mother. It was clear to all of us that she was departing for good this time. After battling lymphoma for eighteen months, my mother had finally run out of lucky breaks. The chemo was not working.

She was back in the hospital. Holmer visited her every day and would jump right into her bed to lie alongside her until the nurses shooed him away so they could take my mother's vitals.

Mom has a point with these signs, I told my sisters as they climbed into the car at the airport. *Very confusing.* It's all about your perspective, we agreed.

Father Wayne, the new, young associate at St. Francis Xavier, was already in my mother's hospital room when the three of us arrived. Holmer, Mary Kay, and our three brothers were gathered there, too.

My mother was too weak to say more than a word or two at a time. *Baby,* she said, pointing to Molly as we walked in the room. With the nine of us assembled, Father Wayne took out his kit with the crucifix, candle, holy water, and oil and started on the last rites.

Jean, you have a lovely family, the young priest said.

My mother looked at each one of us and nodded.

Do I ever, she said.

We held hands and said the Hail Mary.

As we left to get some dinner, Holmer pulled me aside. *I don't want you staying here again tonight,* he told me. *You need to pace yourself.*

Mary Kay had held vigil earlier in the week, and I had slept in a chair in my mother's hospice room for the two previous nights, but I was not about to abandon ship now. Besides, I wasn't going to miss out on the chance to spend time with Patty and Molly.

Okay, Holmie, I told him, promising to let someone else handle overnight duty. *But don't wait up for me.*

My mother's deathwatch felt like a slumber party—three sisters snuggled in cots with our mother watching over us. A good friend of hers from AA stopped by briefly, giving her a kiss on the forehead as she left. My mother had stopped talking altogether early that evening, so, once we finally shut up, the only noise in the room was the humming of her morphine drip and an occasional bit of snoring.

Hey! Pipe down over there, I cried out faintly to my mother, *or I'll beat you to a bloody pulp.*

After a while, each of us drifted off to sleep.

I have never been able to understand how the rest of that night happened the way that it did, so peacefully and perfectly calibrated. Without provocation, I woke up first and went to my mother's side, taking hold of her right hand. It was a little after 2:20 a.m. The blinds were cracked open a bit, letting in a sliver of light from the parking lot. A few minutes later, Patty woke up silently, and she went over to my mother's other side, taking her left hand. Still, no talking. Just the dripping and humming. Molly stirred a few minutes after that, stood at the end of the bed, and began to rub our mother's feet.

Blabbermouths all—especially me—and, still, no one said a word. The three of us stood staring at our mother, watching her chest rise and fall. We hung on her every breath. Up and down. Up and down. Up. And. Down. Then, her eyes opened, fluttering, and she looked around the room, not focused on any of us, just kind of casing the place. We looked at each other. Then back at her. Something was happening, but we weren't sure what. What was she looking for? Who was she looking for? Her chest kept moving. Up. And. Down. She didn't look scared or annoyed. She looked like she was about to leave home, standing at the front door on Greenwood Avenue, and she wanted to take all this in one last time.

We leaned in.

Go in peace, Mommy, Molly whispered.

My mother closed her eyes, and, after a few more breaths, her chest lay still. We waited. Nothing. And waited. Still nothing. The three of us stood there in a kind of a glow. We felt no anxiety, no tension or sorrow. Just peace, like we had been midwives, ushering our mother gently out of one world and into another. A few minutes later, the nurse came in and took over.

No more mounds of laundry or playground duty on sleety November days. No more reaching for a nip of gin to stop the shaking inside. No more obsessing about how Nancy made it to the train tracks.

Patty and Molly waited until Mary Kay could get to the hospital to say her goodbyes. I drove back to the town house to deliver the news to Holmer.

He was lying there on his side, hugging his pillow, just as he was doing the night I sneaked into their room on Thanksgiving so many years earlier. I knelt at his side and put my hand on his shoulder.

Hey, Holmie, I told him, making sure he was awake.

His eyes opened and locked into mine.

She's gone, I said, nodding.

That's it? he asked, scrambling out of the covers. *That's it?*

Then he threw his arms around me and sobbed.

Oh, God, he said. *What are we going to do now? What are we going to do?*

We waited until morning to let Jake and Billy know. But we could not find Danny. He wasn't answering his phone. The Chicago Bears were playing their first game of the season that day, and someone thought Danny might be heading to Soldier Field.

Maybe we can rent one of those airplane signs and fly it over, Billy said, then launched into a James Cagney voice. *Hey, Danny: Ma's dead.*

When Danny finally surfaced, he took the news the same way he did when he heard that Nancy died. No tears. No hugs. He just nodded, his eyes blinking as he walked away. *That's not right,* I thought. Danny loved my mother.

What the hell is wrong with you? I asked him.

A lot, as it turned out. Much more than we ever feared.

II

The Prodigal Son Returns

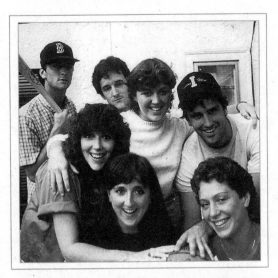

On the patio at our house on Greenwood Avenue.
Wilmette, Illinois, 1984.

We had no clue at the time, but, as our mother lay dying of cancer, Danny was getting into more trouble. A grand jury was about to investigate him. He would be arrested for harassment again.

Danny was still running YardBirds, the lawn care company he started in high school. Despite notoriety from the ugly hate mail incident, he managed to keep most of his customers and added plenty of new ones. By now, he had a few crews of men working for him, a curious mix of old high school pals and men who migrated from Mexico.

But his business was struggling. Danny may have been a fun guy to go to the bars with, but his skills as a boss were sorely lacking. He was woefully disorganized and got flustered easily. He had big dreams but little patience for the intricacies of his business. If customers were late paying their bills, Danny would call to berate them. If they missed two payments, he threatened to take them to small claims court, even if the bill was for as little as eleven dollars. After one customer fired him, Danny had his crew show up on the job anyway and then sent another bill.

That fall, one of his former customers reported to the police that Danny was harassing her multiple times a day on the telephone. Police in Kenilworth, well familiar with Danny from the Weiss Tire case, considered him to be a jerk and a troublemaker. They got a subpoena for his phone records and found that he called the woman fifty times in a twenty-four-hour period, including one call that came in at 4:30 a.m. His explanation: *I can't sleep because of all the money you owe me, so why should you?*

Not long after my mother's funeral, Danny was arrested and charged with harassment. Somehow, his lawyer was able to get the charges dropped, but Danny's mania was intensifying.

From what we could see, Danny was doing reasonably well. In the ten years since his hate mail trial, he transferred to Loyola University in Chicago, where he earned a bachelor's degree in political science and started work on an MBA all while continuing to manage his lawn service. He got a job as a salesman at a Downtown corporate firm but hated the office politics and working with "a bunch of phonies." After a few months, he went back to his landscaping business. He was living in an apartment in Rogers Park, a blue-collar neighborhood Danny cheekily called "Park Roget" hoping the French accent would make it sound more exclusive. He wore a Boston Red Sox cap and surrounded himself with guys a few years younger than he was.

Danny loathed social climbers. He proudly called his group "the Misfits," because, he said, their accomplishments seemed to fall short of the success that many of his North Shore contemporaries enjoyed with their steady girlfriends, corporate jobs, and fancy cars. Danny and his pals played softball and hung out in his apartment, drinking beer, quoting *Caddyshack,* and listening to music, mostly Neil Young, Buddy Guy, and Howlin' Wolf.

He tried his hand at romance without much success. For a while, he had a girlfriend who lived in Wisconsin, but it ended badly. Occasionally, he and Billy would find themselves at the same bar. Debonair as Billy was, he never had trouble attracting a crowd. Danny tried to work that to his full advantage. *Ladies,* Danny would lean in and tell a group of women, pointing across the bar to his older brother. *If you like him, you're gonna LOVE me.* But Danny never felt like he measured up.

His hair was too wiry. His five o'clock shadow too thick. He was too pale and too skinny to be taken seriously. These were all the reasons Danny gave for not getting a girlfriend or a "more respectable" job.

He and his friend Sully bought a clunky used motorboat that they christened the SS *Gilligan.* They would take it out on Lake Michigan on summer nights, cruising the shore as they quoted Monty Python, discussed women they would like to date, and hatched big plans to strike it rich and become famous.

"Danny never felt like he was in the club," Sully told me. "He was always waiting for the next best thing to happen. He'd say, 'Sully, when I get a house, this will all change. When I get a girlfriend, things will be different.' But they never were. He was never content with who he was or where he was in life."

Danny was beginning to realize that his angst was more than the typical insecurities of a person in his late twenties. Deep down inside, he knew something was not right. He was unable to control his emotions. His moods would swing from fits of euphoria—feeling like he was the king of the universe—to black holes of depression, anxiety, and outright panic. By the early 1990s, Danny's friends were growing weary of him. He was wearing them out.

They started noticing how oddly Danny was behaving. He was irritable and erratic, getting in fights with his customers, doing a poor job of keeping his financial records in order. He spent hours in the bathtub, conducting his business by phone, refusing to go outside of his apartment. Sometimes, he wouldn't leave the apartment for days.

"At the time, I just thought it was weird," his longtime friend Mike

Plumb told me years later. "I can see now that he was getting too paranoid to go outside."

I saw what I wanted to see and didn't know how sick he really was becoming. We were swept up in the sadness of losing our mother. It was easier to imagine that Danny was doing well, even though we all had nagging doubts. Mary Kay and I were busy raising our kids, and Molly and Patty lived far away. Danny rarely came around for family gatherings and holidays. When he did, he was very guarded about what he would say, keeping his remarks limited, usually to dialogue from movies like *Spinal Tap* and *It's a Wonderful Life*. He did a pitch-perfect Jimmy Stewart. *You sit there and you spin your little web,* Danny would say to whatever baby niece or nephew we plopped on his lap. *In the whole vast configuration of things, I'd say you're nothing more than a scurvy little spider.*

His comedy routines kept us from seeing how sick he was becoming. We all urged Danny to move to another city, make a fresh start where he wouldn't be hounded by upsetting memories. But he didn't want to talk about it. Whenever the conversation turned the least bit serious, Danny would walk away.

Come out to Utah, Molly pleaded. *You'll be amazed how restorative it is to sleep under the stars.* She sent him a book of prayer, meditation, and spiritual exercises—hoping that it would give him the encouragement he needed to start a new life somewhere else. Patty had stationery made for him with his YardBirds logo, wanting him to see how proud she was of him. He sent it back to her, unopened.

Our cousin Heidi moved to Chicago after college in 1989, and she and Danny got together occasionally for beers, a concert, or a Cubs game. "He really liked my friends," Heidi said. Heidi and her younger brother, George, four and six years younger than Danny, idolized him when they were young. He called them the "easy-living Lutherans" (they weren't Lutherans) and teased them about their stately lake home with its huge white pillars and wraparound porch, saying, *You've got to be really good at cheating on your taxes to live in a place like this.*

Slowly, Heidi observed that Danny had changed from the amusingly whimsical, if impertinent, role model to someone much more menacing. She was mortified when she and her date went to Second City, a comedy club, one night and the guy onstage was pretending to be the neighborhood lunatic, a character named Danny Kissinger.

She would soon find out how Danny had earned that reputation. He had helped her move into a new apartment, lugging a few pieces of her furniture in his truck. She repaid him with a few nice dinners, but Danny started calling her, demanding money. Then he rode past her apartment on his bike, yelling at her through the window. Next, he left angry, menacing messages on her answering machine. Alarmed, Heidi called Holmer to see what she should do. *Just ignore him,* Holmer said.

After he graduated from college, Danny's *Gilligan* cocaptain Sully moved to California to help launch a tech start-up. Not long after he got there, Danny came to visit. Sully was disturbed to learn that the real purpose of Danny's trip was not to see his old pal but to hunt down a former customer to try to get the man to pay his bill.

"Danny thought every customer was out to screw him," Sully said.

We knew none of this. We pretended Danny's problems were behind him; we didn't have the energy to deal with more trouble. By the late summer of 1994, we could not ignore it any longer. Danny came to visit me in Milwaukee, and while he and I were walking along the shores of Lake Michigan, he told me how he sometimes thought about hanging himself. Every once in a while, he tied a rope around his neck or put a bag over his head, *just to see what that feels like.*

His confession knocked the air right out of me. I fumbled for the right words to say to him. Just as I had blown it with Nancy when she would talk about wanting to die, I didn't know what to tell Danny. Even then, all those years after Nancy's death, I did not know how to have a conversation about this. I didn't know that when someone tells you that they have a plan for how to kill themselves, they are in imminent danger. I thought, wrongly, that encouraging Danny to talk about his fantasies of suicide would make him want to act on them even more. I didn't understand then that it could have helped to let him talk about how he was feeling, that sometimes you have to let uncomfortable conversations continue.

It was another lost opportunity. With hindsight, I wish I had said, *I am sorry that you are feeling this lonely. You can get through this tough time. I will help you. We all will. You are not alone.* But I was scared. So, instead, I punched him in the arm and said, *Cut it out.*

Getting Danny to see a psychiatrist would be a real battle. He vehemently denied he needed help and refused to consider medication. In Danny's world, people weren't mentally ill, just weak. He never properly grieved Nancy's death. None of us had. But Danny always seemed especially injured by it. He was embarrassed and angry. He never spoke about her to his friends.

That night, after Danny left, I called Patty to talk about what we should do. She volunteered at a suicide crisis line, and I thought she might have some ideas.

Oh, boy, Patty said.

Over the following week, she and I managed to convince Danny to tell a doctor about his thoughts of killing himself. Not surprisingly, the doctor diagnosed Danny with bipolar disorder and prescribed Paxil, an antidepressant. *Be sure to tell them our family history,* I told Danny more than once. Family members of people who die by suicide have a higher risk of killing themselves. So are those who've spent time in jail. So Danny was considered especially vulnerable.

But a few weeks later, he stopped taking the medication. He said he didn't need it and lashed out at anyone who suggested that he go back on the antidepressant.

I'm not crazy, Danny said. *You are, and so are these doctors.*

I'D CALL TO CHECK in on Danny from time to time, but there is only so much you can do over the phone and only so much Danny was willing to share with me. Even from a distance, I could tell he was growing sicker and more paranoid.

Danny became convinced that he was suffering from a condition called *hyperinsulinism,* which he said clouded his thinking. He had his blood tested, and the results came back normal. It was a delusion. Still, Danny claimed that a fasting plasma glucose test showed a "dramatic fall" in his levels between hour two and hour three of the test, and, in his mind, this confirmed that he had a serious case.

As we saw during his Weiss trial days, Danny was a champion denier. If he dug in his heels hard enough, he thought, he could avoid the reality of his illness. Now he had found a way to describe his behavior in a way that was much more acceptable to him than the truth.

Jake would listen to Danny talk for hours about his blood sugar levels. So would Mary Kay, whose oldest son, Ryan, was diagnosed with diabetes when he was three years old. Danny would stop by her house to show her his blood sugar scores.

He created a handout for all of us, eight pages, stapled together with his picture on the cover and the words *Pre-Diabetic Hyperinsulinism* in huge letters. He included copies of his blood tests and printed out the symptoms of low and high blood sugar, all ailments he reported feeling: irritability, anxiety, pale complexion, confusion, lack of focus or motivation, feelings of "going crazy, even his involuntary blinking." He talked about this to anyone who took the time to listen.

One of Sully's sisters ran into Danny on the commuter train from Chicago to Evanston. *Good news,* he told her. *I finally figured out what was wrong with me after all these years.* Then he handed her a copy of his report. *Everyone said I was crazy,* Danny told her. *I'm not crazy. I'm sick. And here's the proof.*

By September 1995, Danny's lawn business was barely sustainable. He moved to a more affordable apartment in a rougher part of the city. Before long, he was convinced that the next-door neighbors were dealing cocaine from their porch steps, and he reported them to the police. When the cops failed to act to Danny's satisfaction, he sent a notice to all his neighbors, naming names. Then the real trouble began.

Danny said he could hear the drug dealers talking about him through the window, saying things like, "We're going to have to kill him" and

"His ass is mine." He started carrying a baseball bat with him wherever he went. In early October, Danny came across three of the neighbors in the parking lot and started swinging the bat at them. One of them tackled Danny, but he broke free and ran to his truck to grab another bat. They called the police, who arrested Danny and charged him with aggravated assault. Now, Danny was convinced that the cops were conspiring with the drug dealers and only arrested him to shut him up.

More trouble soon followed. A few weeks later, Danny was driving down the street in his truck when he saw a man he thought had given him some trouble at a bar the year before. Danny, a beanpole at six foot one and 143 pounds, pulled his truck over, walked over to the man, and punched him in the nose. Danny ran back to the truck, but the man, bleeding, tackled him. He turned out to be an off-duty Chicago cop. Danny was arrested again, this time for assault and battery, both felonies.

At this point, even Holmer acknowledged that Danny was sick and needed a lot more care than we could give him.

This is fantastic news, I told Holmer when he called to tell me that Danny had been arrested. *Now he'll finally get the help he needs.* That's how desperate we were. We were relieved that he had been arrested and charged with two felonies.

Out on bail, Danny sold his lawn business, and Holmer was paying his rent. In his apartment all day with nothing to distract him, Danny ruminated on how his life had become such a mess. He was angry and bitter, wondering why no one could see how sick he was.

As he awaited trial on the assault charges, Danny turned his attention to his previous legal problems. He began writing menacing letters to Nicholas Pomaro, the judge who had sentenced him to four weekends in jail for the hate mail campaign fourteen years earlier when Danny was a freshman in college. Danny was searching for a way to explain his behavior that he thought would make him more sympathetic. He grew up watching Nancy and Jake and my mother suffer from their depression and anxiety, and he was frantically trying to come up with an alternate explanation for what was happening to him.

In his postcards, Danny claimed to be on a mission from God. His job was to exact justice, he said. He must now become an agent for the truth. If he could not avenge the wrongdoers, he could at least put them on notice that one mightier than he would. "God is watching," Danny warned the judge in the first of his missives. "To conceal the truth is to lie. God and man abhor lies."

He went on for a bit about the medical condition that he was convinced he had. Danny said he was "a sick boy used as a stooge," and this disease had harmed him all his life: "Would all of these bad things (jail, financial loss, hostility, etc. etc.) have happened to me if I wasn't diabetic etc. NO!"

Then came this heartbreaking insight.

"Nobody likes me or wants to be my friend," Danny wrote.

The more he thought about these perceived injustices, the angrier he became. "I would much rather let you continue to make an ass of yourself in front of God and man. In fact, I find it quite enjoyable," Danny wrote. "But I am mandated to divulge the truth or I will have to face the wrath of God and I don't have the strength to get up and take another shot. Lies, deception, fraud, greed, pretension and ambition and abuse is all yours. I wouldn't want to be in your shoes . . . I can rest at night knowing that I am at peace with God and man. Can you?"

Understandably alarmed, the judge called the police, who went to Danny's apartment one Sunday morning in March 1996 and told him to stop sending the letters or they would arrest him for harassment. Danny sent one more, castigating the judge, ironically, for harassing him, and then he stopped.

When his campaign failed to elicit the response he was hoping for, Danny filed a complaint against the judge with the Illinois Attorney Registration and Disciplinary Commission. He claimed the judge had stolen his money, defamed his character, and deprived him of "any fairness." He demanded an investigation.

The police called Holmer to tell him about Danny writing those letters and to check out Danny's claim that he had diabetes. Was that true?

"Yes," Holmer lied. And sometimes, that caused Danny to have "irrational neurological problems," he said.

A few days later, Holmer got a call from Charles Nicodemus, a longtime crime reporter, who had covered Danny's 1982 trial for the *Chicago Sun-Times*. Danny was calling Nicodemus to try to get him to write a story about his blood sugar levels and how he was framed.

"This is like Watergate in reverse," Danny told the reporter.

Because Danny's messages were so rambling and frequent, Nicodemus alerted the lobby guard at the newspaper office and asked him not to admit Danny to the newsroom if he showed up. They posted Danny's picture at the guard station.

Holmer asked me to call Nicodemus, reporter to reporter, to let him know that my brother was sick and that we were working to get him some help. Nicodemus was direct but very nice. "Sorry for all the trouble your family has been through," he said. But that wasn't the end of it.

Nicodemus called me back several weeks later to let me know that Danny had begun calling him again and that the nature of his messages was now "alarming." "It's obvious that your brother's mental condition has deteriorated significantly in the fourteen weeks since we last talked," he said. Danny was angry that Nicodemus had not exposed the judge's alleged wrongdoing. He chastised the reporter for his "irresponsible" and "unethical" reporting in 1982 and told him, "God is angry at you and your newspaper." Then he added, "The place is going to burn, and you'll burn with it." *The cops will be investigating,* Nicodemus told me. *Tell your dad to expect a call.*

Holmer broke down in tears when I told him what Nicodemus reported to me. *Everything's falling apart for him,* Holmer said, sobbing. He said Danny was moving back home so he could take care of him.

That's not a good idea, I told Holmer.

Well, who the fuck do you suggest does? Holmer shouted.

I suggested a halfway house, where trained staff could help Danny get stabilized on his medication.

My naivete amazed Holmer. *Do you really think the state is going to play nursemaid to your brother? They don't give a shit about him.*

Even if he could find such a place, Holmer was not going to subject Danny to the care of strangers. He had seen the conditions at the state hospital where Nancy stayed for a time in 1976, and he was determined not to have another one of his children treated like that—forcefully drugged, dismissed as a problem. Families take care of each other. His children would always have a home to come to if they needed it badly enough.

That's the deal Jake had. Except for the time that he was away at college, Jake always lived at home. "Once a parent, always a parent," Holmer wrote in a little autobiography for his grade school's fortieth reunion.

Jake aspired to a career in international trade, but his depression made full-time work and living independently impossible for him. Some days, it was a chore for him just to get out of bed. We always assumed he would live with Holmer and my mother forever. Jake had a nice group of friends and a sweet girlfriend he saw twice a week. But he never talked about wanting to move away from home, and my parents never encouraged him to.

After my mother died, Jake was a great comfort to Holmer. Thoughtful and kind, Jake helped Holmer around the house, watering the lawn, fixing leaky toilets and dripping faucets. For the most part, he knew how to steer clear of Holmer's tirades.

But Danny, with his fierce temper, was a different story. Holmer was hardly in a position to manage Danny's care. He had his own mental health to tend. To no one's surprise, Holmer had been diagnosed with bipolar disorder a few months after my mother died. He went on a business trip to Kansas City, his first since her death, and while he was standing in line to board his plane, he and the guy in front of him exchanged words, about what, I do not know. Whatever it was made Holmer angry enough that he punched the guy, and the airport police swooped in. We all wrote it off as a reaction to his grief. Then he did it again a few months later, this time to a guy who honked at him at a red light. Holmer threw the car into park and marched back toward the other car. When the man rolled down the window, Holmer leaned down and punched the guy in the face. The

cops arrested Holmer but released him without charging him if he promised to seek medical help. Holmer's doctor prescribed antidepressants and
a mood stabilizer.

Nothing I could say was going to dissuade Holmer from taking Danny
in. He moved into the guest room across the hall from Holmer's bedroom. Jake was sleeping on a bed in the basement. Three wounded bach-
elors would be watching out for each other.

DANNY PLEADED NOT GUILTY to punching the cop, holding fast to his
theory that he was sick, not criminally negligent. He was still unwilling to
consider that his impulsive and erratic behavior was due to mental illness.

"My family wants me to go on lithium but they are nuts," he wrote
to his lawyer, my old high school friend Mike Byrne. My mother was on
lithium for years for her anxiety. We hoped it could help Danny, too.
"Mike, I am sick, not nuts. My father and family do not understand. I can
only say that my disease is totally to blame for all of my legal problems."

The court psychiatrists who examined Danny concluded that he was
not competent to help in his own defense. Danny was delusional and
paranoid, they said. He was not dangerous enough to be committed, but
he should be required to be in treatment and take medication so that he
could be restored to competency. When Danny failed to appear for subsequent sessions, the judge ordered him to be committed to the jail's psychiatric hospital in Elgin until further notice. Once again, I was relieved,
hopeful that now he'd get some good psychiatric care. *This is good news,*
I told Holmer, trying to cheer him up. *They will get him on medication.*

Danny was digging a deeper and deeper hole for himself. We couldn't
imagine how he would ever be able to climb out.

Holmer choked back tears as he told me what happened in court that
morning.

He looked like a wounded deer.

Holmer followed the deputies as they drove Danny to Elgin Mental
Health Center, the psychiatric hospital for the Cook County jail, about
an hour west of Wilmette.

Despite our hopes that Danny would finally get the medical attention he needed, he refused medication and treatment, and no one at the jail's hospital compelled him to try. Holmer was right. No one seemed to give a shit.

Clinical notes I obtained through an open records request decades later show that Danny claimed, incorrectly, that this was his first hospitalization. He said he had never been arrested before and that he had never had thoughts of suicide. When the admitting doctor asked Danny about his family mental health history, he said we had an uncle with bipolar disorder (no idea who this might be) but made no mention of Nancy's suicide or Jake's depression or my mother's depression or Holmer's bipolar diagnosis.

Over the next few weeks, I tried to call Danny at the hospital, but he refused my phone calls. I wrote to him, but my letter came back unopened. The goal was to restore him to competency so that he would be sane enough to stand trial and aid in his own defense. But Danny, convinced he was being railroaded by the system, continued to refuse to take medication or participate in therapy. August gave way to September and then October. They couldn't hold him forever.

In mid-October, the jail staff called Holmer asking if he would allow Danny to live with him once he was released. Danny was still facing the felony assault charges, but he likely would be free while the trial was pending. He needed to live somewhere. Holmer began going to meetings for family members of those being held in the jail hospital, learning about how to care for their relatives once they were released.

I was so angry, I fired off a letter to the judge, signed by all the siblings, to let him know how appalling and highly irresponsible we found this to be.

"The idea of a man, found by two psychiatrists to be legally insane just five months ago—who has not been treated for his illness—living with our father, a 70-year-old widower, is scary indeed," I wrote. Scarier still when that seventy-year-old widower is also bipolar.

Then, in words that would prove to be tragically prescient, we ended the letter by saying, "We are frightened about what might happen if Dan is released without treatment and sent to live with our father."

The judge never acknowledged my letter. Two weeks later, for reasons that are still unclear to me, Danny agreed to take Depakote, a mood stabilizer for people with mania. The hospital social worker reported that Danny continued to insist that his problems were not related to mental illness but caused by his erratic blood sugar levels. But if this was the only way to get out of the jail hospital, he was willing to do it. Since taking the medication, Danny was more cooperative with staff and seemed more relaxed, the social worker noted.

Danny was released on December 20, 1996, four months and five days after he was first locked up. As a condition of his release, he agreed to keep taking the Depakote and attend weekly therapy sessions. Despite my entreaty that Danny be placed in a more therapeutic setting, he was sent home to live with Holmer and Jake.

Danny and Holmer came up to Milwaukee for Christmas Eve dinner with Larry, me, the kids, and Patty, who flew in from New Orleans. *The prodigal son returns,* said Danny with a wide, happy grin as he walked in our front door. Then he turned to us all and uttered his favorite line: *How can I help you when I'm insane?*

Patty shot me a look, and we both rolled our eyes.

Hoo, boy, she whispered. Two weeks later, Danny stopped taking his medication.

12

Collecting Treasures for Heaven

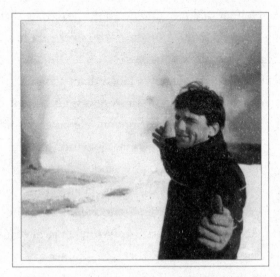

*Danny at Niagara Falls, on his way home from a Loyola
basketball tournament in Rhode Island, 1985.*

Danny never sent me mail. Not a Christmas card. Not a birthday
card. No "Congrats on Your New Baby Girl" or "Thanks for
the awesome Pink Floyd CD." So, when a letter from him arrived in August 1997, I was nervous.

Not only had he stopped taking the medication when he came home
after four months in the jail's psychiatric hospital, but he refused to talk
to his court-ordered therapist. He showed up for the sessions but just
sat there "selectively mute." The therapist threatened to report Danny's
insubordination to the judge, meaning he could be headed back to jail.

Danny was still vehemently resistant to and offended by any suggestion that he had a mental illness. Holmer tried signing him up for disability insurance benefits, but Danny refused to sign the paperwork. He tore up the forms and tossed them into the trash.

Then, around June, with the threat of being locked up again looming, Danny agreed to go back on medication. It was a new one—risperidone, an atypical antipsychotic found to make people less irritable. *It's knocking him on his ass,* Holmer told me, giddy with the possibility that his son was finally getting better. *Good,* I thought. *We'd rather have him a little loopy than angry and agitated.* If only I knew.

The risperidone changed Danny's mood dramatically. Long known for his cynicism and smart-ass remarks, Danny now seemed meek, contrite, and preoccupied with the notion of redemption. He began reading the Bible, making lists of ways to be a better person. He started going to Bible studies at an evangelical church where they talked about false prophets and the need to surrender to God's will. He asked Jake and Holmer to pray over him. We found this hyper-religiosity unsettling, but if the medication was helping Danny come to terms with his illness, we were all in favor of him taking it.

The letter that Danny sent me that late-summer day wasted no time getting right to the point:

Dear Meg,

I wanted to let you know how truly sorry I am for my behavior over, really, the last year or years. I had no idea how bad I was behaving and that my ways were truly sinful and wrong. I know that I am bipolar and that this is a really awful disorder which makes me think awkwardly and I get caught up in foolish ways. Please accept my apology and I will continue with medicine and therapy. I was the last person to know how sinful and ignorant I was, and it has cost me dearly.

At first, I was blown away. This didn't sound like the Danny Kissinger I knew. I read his letter over a few times to let the words sink in. It lacked his usual sarcasm. There was none of his usual defensiveness and anger. He was asking for forgiveness. His words were generous and humble.

Having once been so cruel and dismissive of others not like him, Danny seemed to be learning humility. He appeared to grasp to it. Was this the real Danny, finally free from the shame he'd felt for so many years?

I always thought that his biting, sometimes cruel demeanor had been a defense mechanism, a way to hold us at arm's length so we couldn't see how sick he really was. Now, studying his words, I started to have hope that Danny was forgiving himself and asking others to forgive him so that he could get his life together. He could build himself back up again, the way Holmer and my mother had done once they finally kicked their alcohol dependencies. It wouldn't be easy—Danny was still in a lot of trouble legally and financially—but it was a start.

Maybe the medication cleared away the cobwebs in Danny's head, giving him a clarity and insight that he couldn't have before. Danny went into great detail in his letter about what it was like for him to have bipolar illness and how people need to understand that it is a sickness, not a choice.

"Only love and understanding can conquer this disease," he wrote.

The more I thought about this, the more I began to worry. The tone was off. This seemed to me to be too drastic of a change in attitude. All this talk about sinfulness was making me nervous. There was a kind of finality to the way Danny worded his letter that made me uncomfortable. He sounded like someone who just came out of a stupor, taken inventory of his life, and realized that he screwed it up beyond repair. He was saying goodbye, but before he left, he wanted to leave a legacy, a kind of prescription for how to help others. *Only love and understanding can conquer this disease.*

I thought about the way my mother looked just before she died, how she scanned the room, taking one last look around. That's what Danny's letter seemed like to me. He was looking around and saying goodbye. I started to panic.

Oh my God, I thought. *This is a suicide note. Danny's going to kill himself.*

I ran to the phone to call Holmer.

Where is he? I demanded.

Settle down, Holmer answered. *He's in the next room sleeping.*

Go in there and check. Now! I was frantic.

So, Holmer did. And Danny was fine. But I still couldn't shake the feeling that something was terribly wrong. I read about how people who go on medication can become suicidal once the drugs start to work. They finally have the clarity of thought and the energy to do the only thing they think will help. The medication Danny was taking was known to increase thoughts of suicide in some patients.

Please watch out for him, I told Holmer.

Billy was worried, too. On the same day that I received my letter, Danny had left a message for Billy on his answering machine apologizing for being such a jerk to him over the years. *You've been a good brother to me,* Danny said. *I love you.*

At first, Billy, like me, was touched that his younger brother seemed to be making amends. But the more Billy thought about it, the more he came to the same conclusion. Billy was spooked. He, too, feared that Danny was suicidal.

Holmer and Danny were planning to come up to Milwaukee the following Friday for our annual Irish music festival. This would be a chance for me to see for myself how Danny was doing. But Holmer called that Friday morning and said Danny wasn't feeling well. They would try to come up in a day or two.

I WAS IN THE newsroom the next day, a Saturday, scrambling to finish a story, when my phone rang.

Hey, Holmer said.

I thought he was calling to tell me what time he and Danny would be arriving that day, but his voice sounded winded. He was panting, like he had been running.

Is someone there with you? Holmer asked. I could tell by the tone of his

voice that something was very wrong. My heart started to pound. I took
a deep breath.

Why? I said, trying not to panic. *Where's Danny?*

Long pause.

Where is he? Now I was standing at my desk screaming, and the assistant metro editor came over to see what the matter was. He put his hand
on my shoulder. *Where is Danny?*

He's dead, Holmer sobbed. Jake had found him with a cord around his
neck at the bottom of the basement stairs. *The cops are down there with
him now.*

The room began to spin, and I felt my knees buckle. The editor
grabbed me by my shoulders and helped me into my chair.

This can't be happening, I said. Now I was panting. *How can this be
happening? It can't be. We can't do this again. No!*

I walked up and down the hallway off the newsroom, trying to collect
myself.

A few minutes later, I called Larry and told him the news, then asked
him to go get the kids, who were swimming in our town pool with some
friends. Charley was eleven years old, and Molly was ten. They were still
in their wet bathing suits when I walked in the door about twenty minutes later. They knew I had an older sister named Nancy who died many
years earlier and that she ended her own life. I had done my best to paint
her as a real person to them over the years, someone they did not need to
fear. They heard me tell stories about the time the two of us got caught in
the bowling pin reset machine in a hotel in St. Louis and how she had a
mole on her left wrist that we used to call her "tickle button." Still, Nancy
was an invisible character to them, like Uncle Jack had been to me, more
of an idea than a real person.

But they knew Danny. He was the goofy uncle who would give them
rides in his wheelbarrow. We always laughed about the time I was trying
to get two-year-old Charley to take a nap and Danny interfered, telling
him, *You're a man now, son, don't let your mother boss you around like this.*

How do you tell kids that someone in their family is dead because he killed himself? How do you talk about suicide without normalizing it or vilifying it? I did not want them to think this was a logical, acceptable solution to Danny's problems. But I didn't want them to be frightened when they thought about him either. And I certainly wasn't going to pull a Holmer and say, *If anyone asks, this was an accident.*

There was no time to consult a child psychologist or even their pediatrician. I was anxious to get down to Wilmette as quickly as I could to be there for my father and Jake. I knew I had Larry there to be the rock. He would let them watch Nickelodeon and make sure they were in bed with their teeth brushed by eight o'clock. We would have plenty of time later to let the school know and get them into counseling.

Uncle Danny died today, I told them, *because he did not want to be alive anymore.* They nodded and blinked. Ten minutes later, I was on the road.

Father Klein, one of the priests at St. Francis, was sitting in the living room when I walked into Holmer's town house. The police had just left.

The story I pieced together about how Danny died comes from Holmer, Jake, and records I eventually got from the Wilmette police: Danny was sleepy that Friday from his new medication, so he didn't come downstairs for dinner, not even after Holmer went upstairs to try to convince him to eat something. Holmer got up early the next morning to play golf, and as he walked past Danny's bedroom at around 7 a.m., he noticed that Danny was still asleep. Jake was staying at his girlfriend's apartment, so Danny was home alone.

Holmer returned at around 1:30 that afternoon and started making lunch in the kitchen when Jake and his girlfriend, Annie, walked in the back door. The three of them made small talk for a few minutes, and Jake went downstairs to get something from his bedroom. As he started down the stairs, Jake could see Danny slumped on his knees.

He called out to Danny.

No answer.

Then he saw the cord around Danny's neck. When Jake realized what had happened, he screamed so loudly that Annie hurried down the stairs.

As Jake frantically searched for wire cutters or some scissors, Annie called 911. Holmer scrambled down and found Jake searching Danny's wrist for a pulse. They took turns trying to revive him with mouth-to-mouth resuscitation. The police arrived less than ten minutes later, but it was too late. Danny hadn't been dead long. His abdomen was still warm.

ONCE AGAIN, IT DIDN'T take long for the house to fill up. Word had already spread to St. Francis, and by the time the 5 p.m. Saturday Mass was over, everyone there knew that Danny was dead. The casseroles and plates of cookies and bottles of Scotch started piling up on the dining room table. Mary Claire made a beeline from Communion to Holmer's. *Not Danny,* she said, standing in the doorway, tears spilling down her cheeks.

Putting on a funeral takes lots of planning: the wake, the casket, picking out songs for the service, readings, lining up pallbearers, what to wear, whom to feed and how. My mother wasn't there anymore to see to those details. Instinctively, I pulled out my reporter's notebook and started making one of her famous to-do lists.

Which funeral home do you want me to call this time? I asked Holmer. There were two in our town that catered to Catholics. We used one for Nancy and another for my mother.

Let's go back to Donnellan, he said. *I like to spread the business around.*

The priest encouraged Holmer to wait to schedule the wake and funeral, to give us time to let this sink in and deal with it thoughtfully. But Holmer wanted to get it over with as quickly as he could. The wake would be on Tuesday and the funeral on Wednesday.

Patty and Molly flew in the next day. Once again, I drove to the airport to fetch them.

We've got to stop meeting like this, Patty said as she slid into the passenger side, and we all wiped away our tears.

Holmer insisted on an open casket this time.

He was such a good-looking kid.

So we crossed our fingers and hoped that we wouldn't be able to see the bruises on Danny's neck from where the electrical cord dug in.

In the nineteen years since Nancy's death, the Catholic Church had softened its position on funeral Masses and burials for people who died by suicide. Each bishop was left to decide whether to grant a funeral mass and allow burial in holy ground. Luckily for us, the Archdiocese of Chicago was more progressive than most when it came to ministering to families of those who killed themselves.

We let the priest give the eulogy this time. None of us had the energy or the insight to put our thoughts into words. We were much too raw. There was nothing we could say that would make sense. So no one got up and said what a cute little kid Danny was with his chocolate-brown eyes and crooked smile. Duper, the Dupe, half of the Diapered Duo, the little guy who got stuck in the snow, the Good, Good Baby, the kid who learned how to make BLTs "for Mummy!"

No one said how he tried so hard to bounce back after the awful mess he made with the auto shop owner and how he got his master's degree in business or how he took his workers out on his crummy little motorboat on Lake Michigan on summer nights, collected toiletries and furniture for them and their families. Or how he took in a stray beagle and named the little puppy Old Jack.

But neither did anyone acknowledge that they watched Danny deteriorate from a glib, charming, generous friend to someone most people tried to avoid. By the time he died, Danny, like Nancy, didn't have many friends left. Some of his old high school pals had not seen him in years.

Holmer insisted on playing the Irish ballad "Danny Boy" at the funeral.

The summer's gone and all the roses falling,
Tis you, tis you must go and I must bide.

It was a bit much.

Is he trying to kill us, too? Billy asked as the sound of muffled sobs floated through the pews of St. Francis.

Once again, we trudged up to Milwaukee so Danny could be buried beside Nancy and my mother. No one got lost this time.

Practice makes perfect, Patty said.

Our family language of wisecracks and one-liners had been our way of keeping us all from panicking, to distract us from the truth that we were scared out of our minds. We used humor as a kind of Band-Aid, to keep the fear and anger from infecting us. But wounds also need fresh air and sunlight to heal, and we still weren't ready to sit down as a group and thoughtfully consider what was happening. We were simply in survival mode.

Something clicked with all of us in the months after Danny died. We began to feel cursed. If this could happen twice in our family, why not a third time? Or a fourth? Was there something in our gene pool that would kill each of us? *Our Jean-and-Bill pool,* as we called it. We started looking around, wondering who might be next. Nature or nurture? Either way, we were screwed.

Take two alcoholics—one with bipolar and the other with crippling anxiety—and let them have eight kids in twelve years: What could possibly go wrong?

It was easier to be angry. So, we let Holmer have it. How could he have been so reckless to leave Danny alone that morning?

He couldn't claim that he didn't know that Danny was suicidal. In fact, Danny, like Nancy, relayed a very specific plan to Holmer a few days before he died. He told Holmer that he sometimes walked around the nearby golf course at night surveying which tree would be best for him to hang himself. And, of course, there was the letter that Danny wrote to me the week before and the call that he made to Billy the same day. Still, Holmer would not allow himself to second-guess.

Stinkin' thinkin', said Holmer, employing one of his oft-used AA adages. *No sense in prosecuting the past. It won't change the outcome.*

As far as Holmer was now concerned, it was God's will that Danny was dead, not because he went golfing that morning. Yes, but if you had stayed home then, Danny would not have died, we told him.

Holmer said, *True, Danny wouldn't have died that morning, but what about the next day? Or the next? Or the day after that?*

But we knew Danny was thinking of killing himself, I said. *He told us, for Christ's sake. There must have been more we could have done to stop him.*

There's no sense in what-ifs, Holmer said. *You can't babysit another adult twenty-four-seven for the rest of your life.* Round and round we went.

Even though Holmer was not willing to accept responsibility for Danny's death, he was tortured about what to do with his grief. The bodies were starting to stack up. A dead wife and, now, two dead children. With each new loss, the sorrow seemed to multiply, so that you weren't just mourning one but all three, like they were piggybacking on one another. Holmer started reading the Book of Job for inspiration.

He pored over the passages again and again looking for clues about how to respond to relentless suffering. Biblical scholars consider Job to be the most intense of all the books of the Bible. Job, who lost all he had in one calamity after another, railed against God, wondering why he'd been punished when he was a good man and lived honorably. The message of Job, Holmer learned, is that you need to take life as it comes, surrender completely to the will of God, and trust his judgment. God is not a vending machine, giving prizes for good behavior. Neither is he vengeful, punishing you for being bad.

This was completely contrary to the way Holmer had been raised. Grandma and the nuns with their rosaries and guardian angels and interceding saints had taught him to bargain with God. He grew up believing that if you wanted something badly enough, pray. A new job? Pray! A baby? Pray some more! A cure for your cancer? Say a novena, nine Hail Marys once a day for nine days.

Job's message intrigued Holmer. If we are not punished for our bad behavior or rewarded for the good we do, we might as well live the way we want to, Holmer figured. He interpreted the lesson as a kind of theological "Fuck it."

Holmer resolved not to see Danny's death as a punishment. That fall he went on a silent retreat to a monastery in northern Illinois. (Holmer staying silent for two days? We could not imagine.) At the end of the weekend, the retreatants met with a priest to discuss what they discerned in the silence. Holmer was tired of playing the role of the pitiful loser / sad sack. Enough already with this modern-day Job bullshit.

Goddamn it, Father, Holmer said. *I'm fried.*

Holmer was expecting the priest to give him a lecture about how he needed to work harder to talk to God as Job did. *Faith is like a muscle, Bill,* he thought the priest would say. *You have to work at it if you want it to grow stronger.* But the priest said no such thing. He simply leaned closer to Holmer, put his hands on his shoulders, and whispered, *Be good to yourself, Bill.*

That's it? Holmer asked.

That's it, the priest said.

Holmer started checking out and letting go. He traveled alone to Istanbul to walk along the road to Damascus, where Saint Paul was blinded by the light of Christ. Holmer was hoping for a conversion of his own— one where he would no longer be victim to the cruelties of life.

He didn't seem motivated to order a headstone for Danny. So, I did, but realized too late that I got the year of his birth wrong. I put 1964 when it should have been 1963. These kinds of typos—literally etched in stone—are not easily erased. *Where's the copy desk when you really need them?* I tried to soft-pedal my mistake to Holmer by making a little joke.

I was told there would be no math, I said. *Besides, Danny would think that was funny.*

Holmer wasn't buying it.

Bullshit, he barked back. *You fucked up.*

Yes, I thought. *We all did.*

Even with his new attitude, clearly Holmer harbored some unresolved anger, whether he would admit it or not. A few months later, an agent for the Internal Revenue Service called looking for Danny. Apparently, he owed some money in back taxes.

No, I'm sorry, Dan can't come to the phone, Holmer told the agent. *He's dead right now.*

DON WALKER, A GOOD friend and one of my favorite editors, asked me if I would consider a follow-up to the story I wrote about Nancy ten years earlier. He thought readers would be interested to know how a family copes with the trauma of suicide twice.

Are you out of your damn mind? I told Don. How could I possibly write about something so painful? Why would anyone want to take advice from people stupid enough to let this happen twice? We were losers, as far as I was concerned. *To lose one sibling is a tragedy,* I said, paraphrasing the old Oscar Wilde quote. *To lose two looks like carelessness.* Besides, Danny was hardly a sympathetic character. I'm sure plenty of people remembered his role in the hate mail case and thought Danny had gotten exactly what he deserved.

Then, a few months later, two seemingly unrelated events happened that changed my mind. On New Year's Eve, Bobby and Ethel Kennedy's son Michael was playing football on skis in Aspen, Colorado, when he slammed into a tree and broke his neck, killing himself almost instantly. In a family famous for fast lives and tragic endings, Michael was one of the more notorious Kennedys. He had made headlines years earlier for having sex with his children's fourteen-year-old babysitter. Still, the outpouring of grief from his brothers and sisters was striking.

Like Danny, he'd humiliated his clan. Yet his siblings found the grace to eulogize him so tenderly that it was impossible not to share in their sorrow. His brother Joe called Michael "one hundred points of light" and invoked an A. E. Housman poem, saying his fun-loving spirit was "like the wind through the woods, through him the gale of life blew high."

We loved Danny no less. But this is what suicide does. It deprives families of their primal need to grieve fully. The shame of how they died overshadows them. We don't talk about people we love who end their own lives in the same way that we would if they had died of leukemia or had been killed in a skiing accident. It's an especially lonely kind of grief.

Danny made a mess of his life, but he didn't ask to be sick and, as we soon learned, he was fervently trying to turn things around. While Holmer was in Oregon visiting Molly, Billy and I decided to clean out Danny's belongings. We came across a planner with a list of our names and birthdays. Danny was collecting words of inspiration that he titled "Ways to Live a Better Life." "Do not have thoughts for tomorrow, only today," Danny wrote to himself. "Shine and do good works. Forgive yourself. Collect treasures for Heaven." Was Danny in heaven? Was there a heaven? I sure as hell hoped so.

Billy's shoulders started to shake as we read these notes. We both took deep breaths, hoping the air would steady us. We imagined Danny poring over his self-help books, desperate for instructions, then sitting down and scribbling these bromides in a frantic effort to get well. Now we could see what we hadn't been able to before: Danny was scared and fighting as hard as he could. We'd both read plenty of stories about people with cancer who had battled to the end and what noble warriors they were. How was Danny's campaign any less heroic?

Maybe Don, my editor, was right. Maybe our family's story could help others.

Okay, I told Don. *What the hell. I'll write that story.*

Even Holmer gave his approval. He was so angry when I wrote about Nancy's death years earlier that I wasn't sure how he would react. But in the ten years since then, Holmer saw how people with mental illness are discriminated against, how family and friends get burned out, and how hard it is for people to get care. He knew this was a scandal worth exposing. He had come a long way from *if anyone asks, this was an accident.*

It took me a couple of months to write the story. We had just gotten Bailey, a beagle puppy. I tethered the little guy to a leash around my waist while I wrote, finding the "pet breaks" to be therapeutic. To tell the truth, the story wasn't very well written. Just like the one about Nancy years earlier, it rambled, lacking sharp insight. I was too raw with grief to make much sense. Still, the story resonated with readers. The sheer novelty of it drew a powerful reaction. Even by 1998, people still were not used to these first-person testimonials in their morning newspaper, especially when the subject was mental illness.

So many people called me to talk about the story that my newsroom answering machine maxed out. The clerks collected the overflow of letters in two big plastic bins. It took me weeks to get back to those who called or wrote. Everyone who reached out had heartbreaking stories of their own that they wanted to tell me. A son who hears voices, a daughter who won't eat, a sister who won't leave her bedroom. They told me about their family members who would not admit that they were sick. I heard from people who could not find a doctor who would see them and people whose insurance wouldn't cover treatment and they couldn't afford to pay out of pocket.

The names and many of the details were different, but I quickly picked up on a universal theme: People are frantic to get care for their family members suffering from mental illness. They didn't know whom to call. They were either too embarrassed to talk to anyone about it or they couldn't find anyone who would listen. So, they watched, day after day, while a little bit more of the person they loved disappeared before their eyes. They were confused, angry, and frustrated. But, mostly, they were terrified.

It didn't take long for me to figure out that I had tapped into a rich vein of seemingly endless stories about the failures of our nation's so-called mental health care system, which really is no system at all. I could spend years telling these stories and never run out of page 1 material. My editor agreed.

So that's what I did.

I wrote down a line from Danny's letter on a notepad and taped it to the side of my computer in the newsroom. It became my battle cry.

Only love and understanding can conquer this disease.

As far as I was concerned, Danny summed up everything you need to know in those eight little words. If you love someone, you will try to understand them. You won't turn away.

For the next twenty-five years, I traveled across the country and beyond, looking for the answer to two simple questions: Why are people with serious mental illness so misunderstood, and how can we treat them better? It was too late to help Danny and Nancy. If I was going to understand the illness that killed two of the people I loved most, I would need to look to strangers for answers.

What I found shook me to my core.

PART II

---◆---

Against My Bones

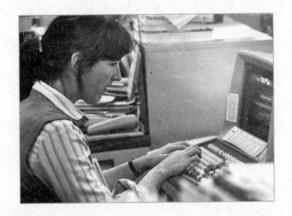

13
Swimming Back to Devil's Island

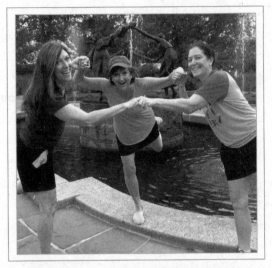

Mary Kay, me, and Patty goofing around at the Three Sisters Fountain, Central Park, New York City, 2017.

In headlines and news copy, we call them "the mentally ill." In truth, they are our mothers and fathers, our brothers and sisters.

They are us.

The National Institute of Mental Health estimates that fifty-three million Americans, or one in five, struggle with some condition that affects their mood, thinking, or behavior. Most have mild forms of mental illness with symptoms that come and go. Often they find relief with medication and therapy.

My focus was on the much smaller subset of this group, the 5.6 percent of adults who suffer from serious and persistent mental illness. Like

Nancy and Danny and Jake, they may be intellectually sharp but have functional impairments that substantially interfere with their ability to take care of themselves. Their thinking is clouded. They get confused easily. They're often overwhelmed. They may have a hard time sleeping, making decisions, holding a job, staying in relationships, making their own meals, paying their bills, and caring for other basic needs. Some are not able to separate fantasy from reality or even recognize that they are sick. Their illnesses are chronic, meaning a lifetime of struggle.

As I plowed through the letters and phone messages that readers sent after my story about Danny's suicide, I learned how people with these crippling illnesses—major depression, schizophrenia, bipolar illness—are cast aside, ignored, even vilified. I knew only too well how we tend to blame them—or their families—for their sickness, as though they brought it on by some moral failure.

We claim to have a mental health system in this country. But that's not true. A system is defined as a "set of things working together," and, as I saw through my reporting and as a family member, very few things work together to help people with mental illness. More than one-third of all people with serious mental illness don't get treatment.

We don't have enough doctors. Many psychiatrists will only treat those who can pay directly. They won't accept Medicare or Medicaid. Even with parity laws, insurance companies won't pay many mental health claims.

People with serious mental illness can't find landlords who will rent to them or employers who will give them steady jobs. A person with serious mental illness is ten times more likely to be incarcerated than hospitalized. Jails and prisons have become the nation's de facto mental health hospital system. The Cook County jail, where Danny spent four months, is now one of three of the largest mental health facilities in the country. More than a quarter of the nation's 559,000 homeless have a serious mental illness. Their average life span is ten to twenty years shorter than the general population.

Yet this kind of prejudice and discrimination is allowed to fester because the aggrieved are either too embarrassed to speak up or we choose to ignore them.

That was the story I wanted to tell: the scandal of how millions of America's most vulnerable people are being abandoned by the very institutions designed to protect them. Government agencies, police, schools, the insurance industry, hospitals and health care providers, even religious organizations, all turn a blind eye to so much of the suffering.

I had no shortage of people willing to tell me how the system had failed them in heartbreaking ways.

Kathy Weigl kept boxes of three-ring binders filled with thousands of pages of documents showing how the army had bungled the care of her son James, a goofy, lovable Iraq War soldier who had two disabling conditions that should have disqualified him from enlisting. When he started to struggle, his supervisor berated him as "weak." When he took a leave of absence after trying to kill himself, the supervisor told the others in James's unit that they'd have to work harder to make up the slack. A year after he was discharged for depression, James hanged himself in his garage.

Helen Kriewaldt would call me drunk, once at 3 a.m., wailing, as she recalled how her son, John, thirty, died after hitting his head in the back of the police squad car on his way to the psychiatric emergency room. "I shouldn't have called the cops on him," she cried. "They didn't know how to handle him right." But what else could she do? John had been out of control that night, throwing furniture around the house. She was too small and thin to stop him, and nothing she was saying would calm him down. "I killed my son," she sobbed.

Yvonne Panetti thumbed through the pages of her son Scott's baby book, looking for evidence of how his life took such a wrong turn. Scott was on death row in Texas, waiting to be executed for killing his in-laws while in a psychotic trance. Scott's wife had tried to turn his guns over to the police the day before, but the officer refused, saying, "Ma'am, a man's guns are sacred property."

"This one turns my blood cold," Yvonne said, pointing to the photo of a five-year-old Scott in a cowboy costume, guns in both hands.

Listening to these mothers and dozens of others was excruciating. But if my reporting was going to show how our institutions had failed them, I'd need to provide the evidence, comb through medical records, sit in their childhood bedrooms, see their Boy Scout badges and homemade Mother's Day cards, and imagine what their lives could have been if they'd gotten the help they needed.

As I traveled across the country, I discovered how my family's struggles were eerily intertwined with pivotal moments in the history of America's fractured mental health system. We Kissingers had come of age just as failed federal reforms were ushering hundreds of thousands of the sickest patients out of institutions and onto the streets. In the name of civil liberty, we traded one outrage—the warehousing of our sickest psychiatric patients in conditions unfit for animals—for another, deserting them to suffer alone.

DEINSTITUTIONALIZATION WAS SOLID public health policy. If only it had worked. Before sedatives were developed in the late 1940s, patients like Danny and Nancy, with extreme forms of mental illness, were housed in large psychiatric facilities, often run by the states, located on the outskirts of town so that no one needed to see or think about them.

But when Thorazine was developed in the late 1940s to battle nausea and allergies, doctors realized that the drug also had a tremendous calming effect. They began using it to sedate patients with psychosis so that they wouldn't need to confine them with straitjackets or shackles. Nor, for that matter, would most of them need to be kept in institutions, unwieldy to manage and expensive to maintain. The federal government began considering alternatives for the more than 560,000 severely mentally ill Americans who were living in psychiatric hospitals.

Not all these institutions were snake pits, of course. But many of them were. For the most part, they were hidden from view until a group of conscientious objectors were assigned as orderlies in state mental hospitals during World War II. The orderlies were shocked at the sight of patients who had been crammed into decrepit, overcrowded quarters, beaten and chained to their beds. Some patients were naked and emaciated, covered in feces or bedsores or both. The orderlies leaked photos to journalists whose exposés described the scenes with graphic precision. Their stories read like pages of gothic horror novels.

Albert Q. Maisel's 1946 *Life* magazine report, "Bedlam," and Albert Deutsch's book *Shame of the States,* published two years later, pulled back the curtain on ghastly, inhumane treatment. The photos recalled images that readers had seen of the people rescued from the Nazi concentration camps just a year or two earlier. Ken Kesey's book *One Flew Over the Cuckoo's Nest,* a fictional account of the cruelties he'd witnessed during his time as an attendant at a state psychiatric hospital in Oregon, came out in 1962, stirring public outrage to the boiling point.

The next winter, President Kennedy, whose sister Rosemary was institutionalized alongside my uncle Johnny in Jefferson, Wisconsin, proposed the Community Mental Health Act of 1963 to federalize mental health care.

"Almost every American family at some stage will experience or has experienced a case of mental affliction," the president said, urging Congress to act. "We have to offer something more than crowded custodial care in our state institutions."

The federal government would take on oversight of people with mental illness from the states so that care could be standardized. The plan was exquisitely simple: divide the country into catchment areas, like mini congressional districts. Each area would have its own mental health authority to oversee the various levels of care. Hospitals would serve the very sickest. Outpatient clinics would be available for those who only needed therapy and their medicines dispensed. Each catchment area would provide community services like classes on coping skills for battling anxiety and wellness checks for new mothers struggling with postpartum depression.

"When carried out, reliance on the cold mercy of custodial isolation will be supplanted by the open warmth of community concern and capability," a smiling Kennedy proclaimed. The bill passed with overwhelming support, 72–1 in the Senate and 335–18 in the House. At last, the era of better mental health care had arrived. Or so everyone thought.

Three weeks later, Kennedy was killed by an assassin in Dallas. The Community Mental Health Act would be the last piece of legislation he would sign. The handsome young president was not all that was lost that day. A great deal of enthusiasm and political momentum for mental health overhaul died with him.

With the public attention now fixed on the assassination, the war in Vietnam, and burgeoning civil unrest, the needs of people suffering from severe mental illness were all but forgotten. Two decades later, Jimmy Carter did his best to restore enthusiasm for reform, championing the passage of a 1980 bill that provided federal grants to community mental health centers. But when Ronald Reagan won the presidential election later that year with the promise of getting the federal government off our backs, his first act was to push for a repeal of the bill, which Congress did.

The onus of care was back in the laps of the states. The states, in turn, foisted much of the responsibilities onto their counties. Funding for mental health care—provided by the federal government and filtered through grants to the states—now had to compete with road repairs, park upkeep, and dozens of other more popular constituent demands for county officials' attention and resources. The quality of public mental health care depended largely on which zip code you lived in.

A tiny band of do-gooders and distraught family members would show up at county board meetings and advocate for the needs of people with severe mental illness. But most weren't willing to say anything at all about the needs of their suffering relatives to even their closest confidants, prejudice against people with these illnesses being what it was.

In the end, fewer than half of the mental health centers pledged by the federal government were ever built. "We blew it," the director of Milwaukee's mental health center told me.

At the same time, more than 93 percent of the treatment beds once available nationwide were eliminated. People with catastrophic mental illness were now left to fend for themselves. Many ended up in jails or prisons or living on the street.

JOHN SPOERL PULLED BACK the branches and showed me his favorite spot to sleep. It's on the east side of a berm overlooking a state highway. "You have to be careful," he told me. "There's a guy around here who will stab you if you piss him off." It was the year 2000, three years after Danny's death, and I was working on a story about the history of deinstitutional-ization. Over the next twenty plus years, I would look to John and others like him to help me figure out how the system had failed them and what we needed to do to provide better care.

There was vomit on John's jeans from a crack binge the night before and a urine stain that hadn't quite dried yet. His jacket was torn, and his fingernails were black from the dirt jammed underneath them. He smelled like rotting apples, cigarette butts, and sour milk. The scar that ran down John's neck was a souvenir from a fight he had thirteen years earlier with his neighbor. The man demanded that John give him his last beer. John refused. In the scuffle, the man pushed John from the second-story window of their rooming house to the concrete slab below. The force of the fall caused John's spleen to burst. His feet were cut to shreds. He spent six months mending.

John talked in a deep, round voice that sounds like a tape recording in slow motion. His jaw was clenched and his steel-blue eyes darted from side to side. John loved the freedom to come and go as he pleased, but this scared his mother, Pat.

"It's nice to talk sweet talk about recovery, but the truth is some people, like John, will never be able to look out for themselves without getting into trouble," his mother told me. Her words struck me as harsh at first, but I knew she was right. I'd seen how John and so many others lived.

"I actually like it outdoors," he said with a slight smile. "The stars are so pretty. But it gets cold."

His teeth were brown from tobacco, cracked and ground down in the back.

"He hasn't brushed his teeth in ten years," his mother said.

John took a drag from his cigarette and considered which was worse: to be in danger, as he was on the streets, or to be held captive in a locked hospital ward.

"Either way, I suffer," he said.

The longer I followed John and others like him, the more I could see the relentless torture of their illnesses and how their families, like mine, suffered alongside them. For every person with severe mental illness, there are dozens of others whose lives are upended by their disease.

Pat and her husband, Joe, had three other children: Joe Jr., a philosophy professor; Margie, a physician; and Joanie, an education specialist. It would be hard to find a more resourceful, loving, and concerned family. Well into her eighties, Pat was one of those who showed up regularly at county board meetings pleading for more funding. She helped found the Milwaukee chapter of the National Alliance on Mental Illness, an advocacy group originally formed to help families navigate caring for their once-institutionalized children and siblings. Each of John's siblings advocated for his needs. Even so, John was in and out of jails and hospitals his whole life.

John died of COVID in January 2021 at the age of sixty-one. If the Spoerls couldn't shield John from the ravages of his mental illness, who could?

I understood their frustration as my own family continued to struggle.

TO TRY TO MANAGE their grief after Danny died, Holmer and Jake began going to meetings of a group called LOSS, short for Loving Outreach to Survivors of Suicide, run by the Archdiocese of Chicago. Billy had suggested it. These were forums for sharing. As you would expect, many choked out painful accounts of how their dear ones had died and what they were doing to get by. Holmer, a veteran of AA's twelve-step meetings, was familiar and comfortable with the format. He knew that to move past your pain, you had to humble yourself, admit that you are powerless, then turn yourself over to a higher power who can fill you up again with strength and hope.

Holmer, now sober for more than twenty years, had served as a sponsor to dozens of people who were trying to "stop boozing." He was setting himself up at these grief support meetings to be that same level of superstar. Ever charming, and by dint of his having two dead children to discuss, Holmer became such a celebrity in his grief group that they nicknamed him "Coach."

To commemorate the group's twentieth anniversary, the leaders made plans to construct a quilt, much like the one in Washington, D.C., in memory of those who died of AIDS. Organizers were hoping to borrow a page from the AIDS community playbook, to put faces to the names of victims, hoping to stir greater attention and more resources toward fighting this scourge.

This LOSS quilt would be constructed from one square for the loved one of every member who had died by suicide.

Mary Kay, a whiz with the embroidery needle, agreed to fashion squares for Nancy and Danny. She stitched their names, their birthdays, and the days they died. Theirs would be two of dozens of squares to be displayed at a reception at the archdiocesan headquarters on Rush Street on a Sunday afternoon in March. Patty and Molly lived too far away to come, but Mary Kay, Billy, Jake, Holmer, and I decided to make a day of it. As we arrived, a pianist was tinkling out soulful tunes, designed to get us in the proper, reverent mood.

The squares were laid out on the table in chronological order from the most recent suicide to those that occurred in 1978, the year LOSS was begun, which also happened to be the year Nancy died. There must have been a hundred squares or more. We stopped respectfully at each one, trying to glean what little backstory we could from the information the families provided. Who were these people? What made them want to die? Here, a cheerleader, just seventeen; There, a cellist, twenty-four. So young. So much life ahead of them. We moved forward, wiping back tears when we got to Danny's square.

Damn it, here we go, I thought, when the man started playing "You Are Mine." That song never failed to reduce me to tears.

I am hope for all who are hopeless.
I am eyes for all who long to see.

As we inched forward along the quilt display, huddled together, nervously making our way toward Nancy's square, Jake stopped suddenly, causing us to bump into one another. *What the . . . ?* Jake leaned in for a closer look. "Our loving grandmother," the square said. "87."

Eighty-seven? Jake said. He couldn't understand why an eighty-seven-year-old lady would bother to kill herself when the end for her was surely near. (Jake is a very concrete thinker.) *Couldn't she just have waited a few years?*

Mary Kay snorted, trying to stifle herself, which only made her laugh harder. Then Billy started in. By the time I caught on to what was happening, the Coach was marching toward us, snapping his fingers, looking quite stern.

These squares, tangible manifestations of precious lives lost, were meant to make us cry. Nancy and Danny were gone from us forever. We needed to feel that sorrow, let the tears flow. But we still would not absorb it. Or we could not. We couldn't stay in the moment and soak in the reality. At least not then. It was so much easier to laugh, to break the tension with some wiseass crack or a joke. Holmer leaned in to shush us with piercing eyes and barked, *Goddamn it! No laughing in the fucking suicide line!*

FOR THE SECOND TIME in his life, the seeds of Holmer's romantic coupling were planted inside a church. He met the woman who would become his second wife on Ash Wednesday. She was a widow, introduced to him by a grade school classmate of Billy's who thought these two suffering souls might find solace in one another. They had their first date that Saturday and were engaged four weeks later. *Why so fast?* I asked, worried at how impetuous Holmer could be, a classic symptom of his bipolar illness. *Maybe she's pregnant,* Mary Kay said. She wasn't. She was a seventy-year-old great-grandmother.

In the ten years since our mother had died, we'd given up on the idea of Holmer remarrying. *Why swim BACK to Devil's Island?* he'd always say. After the wife of one of his friends died, Holmer claimed, *SHE died, and HE went to heaven.* We knew the truth. He missed my mother and was craving a relationship, someone to laugh at his one-liners and listen to his stories.

Holmer had gotten engaged less than a year after our mother died, to one of her best friends, a woman we loved. Our families had grown up together. She was Molly's godmother, and Holmer had been godfather to one of her boys. But to the disappointment of us all, the engagement fizzled. She loved Holmer well enough, but I suspected she felt his volatility, shaky financial circumstances, and the drama of our family was too much to take on.

Now, Holmer was swimming back to Devil's Island with a woman many of us had not even met. We also found it strange that the couple was planning to get married in the splashiest way possible: a gala, dinner, and dancing for a hundred guests, followed by their honeymoon, a week at the Waldorf-Astoria in New York City and a week in Paris.

To complicate matters, Jake had been admitted to Lutheran General Hospital's psychiatric unit that spring, so depressed that he was unable to eat.

Jake had been having an especially hard time since he'd found Danny dead at the bottom of the basement stairs. His doctor thought that now, nearly four years later, Jake likely was experiencing some delayed post-traumatic stress. Jake said he wanted to eat, but every bite made him gag. I wondered if this might be related to Holmer's fast-approaching wedding, but Jake said he doubted that.

A few years earlier, at my urging, Jake had moved to an upstairs bedroom. I didn't think Jake should go to bed each night and wake up each morning twenty feet from the spot of his gruesome discovery. Now that Holmer was getting married, Jake would be moving back down into the basement to give the newlyweds a little privacy.

As the wedding neared, Jake's depression grew more intense. He was weak and dangerously malnourished. Charley and I went to visit him at the hospital one Sunday afternoon, and Jake could barely keep his head up.

Friends and relatives were thrilled for Holmer when they learned about his engagement. After all the sadness he'd been through, Holmer surely deserved the love and affection his new wife could offer. Who could be so cruel as to deny him that?

This wedding sounds mighty fancy, I told Patty.

We knew Holmer didn't have a lot of money. He'd carved out a tidy second career as a lawyer, but his cases were small—house closings, guardianships, speeding tickets our friends had racked up, nothing too lucrative. Every once and a while, a judge would assign him a case as a mediator, which paid a bit more.

Holmer had never been good about staying on a budget. He was too impulsive. My mother had managed to keep a lid on his spending. But when she died, so did his financial stability. We'd seen how shopping made Holmer feel powerful, a bit giddy. It gave him a little something to look forward to, to forget the pain he was feeling, if only temporarily. A week after my mother's funeral, Holmer had the living room furniture reupholstered. The month after Danny died, Holmer bought so many Persian carpets, his condo looked like a showroom.

Even so, we were all taken aback by the scale of this wedding. *White dinner jackets? Paris? The freakin' Waldorf-Astoria?*

Maybe *she's* got a lot of money, Mary Kay said. So, I checked, using some internet sites that I discovered in my investigative reporting training. Nope. She wasn't rich. In fact, debt collectors were after her for failing to pay her bills. *Maybe she thinks Holmer has a lot of dough,* I said.

Well, then, said Mary Kay, *the wedding will also be a surprise party.*

Nervous about this prospective wife who seemed to be as lousy at financial management as Holmer, I asked him to consider getting a prenuptial agreement or set up a trust to protect Jake if anything should happen. He blew me off.

Don't be ridiculous, he said.

Patty and I called Holmer's cousin Joe, hoping he'd take up our cause.

Our request seemed reasonable to us. Can't Holmer just set a little some-thing aside so Jake could afford to stay in the area, a world he's always known and where he feels most comfortable?

I'm not touching that with a ten-foot pole, and neither should you, Joe said. *You girls leave your father alone.* And then he hung up.

Jake got out of the hospital a few days before the wedding, just in time to be fitted for the white dinner jacket he would wear to serve as Holmer's best man. The next week, while Holmer and his new wife were circling the Arc de Triomphe, Jake began moving his stuff back down to the basement.

14

Building Character

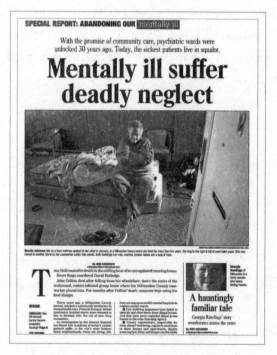

*Inspired by my brother Jake, I spent a year investigating
these stories about abysmal housing in Milwaukee
for people with serious mental illness. (Photo credit:*
Milwaukee Journal Sentinel)

Holmer and his wife didn't technically kick Jake out of the
house. But by 2005, their bills were piling up, and it was looking likely that they would have to sell their three-story condominium and move to a one-bedroom apartment.

There would be no room for Jake in the new place. This would be
trickier than it seemed. Jake, now fifty, had been unemployed for a few

years and was increasingly limited by his depression and anxiety. For more than two decades, Jake worked as a clerk at a neighborhood hardware store—for a man who understood that Jake needed flexible hours to accommodate his lack of energy—but the hardware store had gone out of business, a victim of the big-box industry, and Jake's income was down to his disability check. Even if he could find a place nearby that he could afford on his $540 a month in disability pay, he would have a hard time being on his own. Jake had even more trouble thinking straight. Shopping, cooking, even finding the energy to shower sometimes overwhelmed him. He was nervous about the idea of living alone.

These last five years had been quite a ride for Holmer and his wife. She quit her job shortly after their wedding, announcing that she and her new husband would be traveling the world. The Catholic church where she worked as pastoral director threw a going-away party for her and invited parishioners to send the newlyweds off in style by making donations for her "travel purse."

It felt like a con. We knew they didn't have the resources for world travel. Now, they were passing the plate to have the people of the parish help finance their adventures? I was offended by the idea that some old church lady on a fixed income might feel pressured to donate twenty dollars so Holmer and his wife could visit Via del Corso. Nonetheless, with their travel purse packed, off they went to Italy and Ireland, then Mexico and Hawaii.

Back at home, they ordered catered meals and had fresh flowers delivered each week. They remodeled their kitchen, installing marble countertops, new flooring, and new appliances. Their closets were stuffed with clothes that they charged at Neiman Marcus, Nordstrom, and Saks Fifth Avenue. The bedroom wall was lined with jewelry towers—stacks of earrings, necklaces, bracelets, and rings—and boxes of shoes, including one pair of Ferragamo pumps with a price tag of $750, still wrapped in paper, unworn, months later. Holmer's wife was Imelda to his Ferdinand.

To the outside world, this was a fairy-tale ending—a widower and widow, finally getting to enjoy their golden years with flair after so much heartbreak and loss. As much as I wanted to believe that, too, I knew a grimmer story was developing. They had built their house with matchsticks, and it was sure to blow down any second.

Holmer would call me from time to time to say how nervous he was about how much money the two of them were spending. *We're going to lose this house,* he'd tell me in tears. His wife once picked up the phone from another extension and said, *Bill, this is none of her business.* After that, she stayed on the line each time I called or when Holmer called me.

I was distressed but not sure what I could do to help. I emailed my brothers and sisters, but we all came up clueless about what to do. We weren't going to enable my father and his wife by paying their bills, even if we did have the money. But it pained me to see them getting into trouble. After one especially worrisome phone call, I called Holmer back the next day to see how he was doing, and Jake answered the phone. *They're not home,* Jake said. He had just gotten back from dropping off Holmer and his wife at the airport.

The airport? I asked.

Yeah, said Jake. *They told me not to say anything, but they're in Hawaii for a few weeks.*

It didn't make sense. *How are they going to afford that?* Apparently, on credit cards they knew they wouldn't be able to pay off.

I could somewhat understand why Holmer was letting loose like this. All his life, he had lost so much of what he wanted most—the sailor suit that his mother made him return on the day after Christmas when he was a little boy, his pharmaceutical advertising business with the fancy Fifth Avenue address, the house on Greenwood, his daughter, his wife, his son. He was nearing eighty years old, and his time was running out. So now, he was going whole hog. This was his money. He could do with it as he pleased. If he and his wife wanted to blow every dime, that was their prerogative.

But I also knew that Holmer was sick. His bipolar disorder caused him to lose touch with reality. He'd go on manic spending binges, unable to control himself. He and my mother had bought their condominium with cash in 1990. So it was easy for him to take out a reverse mortgage to pay for these extravagant trips. Now that all the equity was gone, he was borrowing money he no longer had. The credit cards were coming due, and then what? How is it not stealing to be borrowing money you know you don't have and never will? The hypocrisy of the Church Lady and her husband spending money they did not have disgusted me, and I had a hard time hiding it.

Holmer was now facing bankruptcy, and we learned that he and his wife would soon be losing the condo, unable to pay the fees. This didn't just mean an uncertain future for them. It also meant upheaval for Jake, whose home it was, too. We'd all be letting go of a piece of our past. No one had the emotional attachment to the condo the way we did our big Greenwood Avenue home. But at least the condo was common ground where we could gather to hang out as a family, be goofy, bring the grand-kids, gossip a bit, tell funny stories, eat meals off our mother's Wedgwood china, sleep in the bedrooms she decorated with her beloved Waverly floral patterns. Our family had been through so much trauma, we needed ways to keep us together as we continued to heal, someplace that didn't involve a casket or an IV drip.

Little by little, the threads holding our family together were unraveling.

My lifelong pal Mary Claire called me one day from the gym at St. Francis, our old school, where she was helping to run the annual parish rummage sale. She sounded alarmed.

Um, she said, *someone just dropped off boxes of your family's baby pictures. No offense, but no one wants those.* Then she paused. *Well, maybe the frames.*

I knew exactly which ones she meant. They were photos my mother had displayed on the wall leading up to the second floor, pieces of us frozen in time. Mary Kay peacocking in her first pair of high heels, a first-grade Patty squirming in a little nun outfit, Molly proudly holding up six fingers on her sixth birthday. I could understand why Holmer and his wife would want to take down those photos. This was her home now, too. She had seven children of her own, more than a dozen grandchildren, and a few great-grandchildren.

Still, it hurt to think of our family photos being thoughtlessly chucked like a pair of old Moon Boots. Holmer said it was an accident. We sent Jake over to retrieve them, but I couldn't help but be stung by the cruelty of that metaphor.

One family's treasures are another woman's trash.

Later that week, Holmer called to say he and his wife wouldn't be coming up to Milwaukee for our daughter Molly's confirmation ceremony that weekend as planned. Holmer's wife was on the phone line, too. *I've been talking to a woman from church, a psychologist,* Holmer's wife said. *She thinks it would be best for all of us if you kept your distance.*

I was confused. *Why is that?* I asked.

She says that you have inappropriate feelings toward your father.

Wow. So, there it was. *Inappropriate feelings toward your father.* I was so stunned I didn't know what to say. I wasn't going to dignify her accusations with a comment.

I suppose I should have seen it coming. What did I expect? She was angry at how Holmer would call me panicking about the prospect of them having to sell their house to pay the bills. They were both embarrassed they'd gotten themselves into this jam. It was easier to gaslight me than own up to their own reckless acts. Jake and Mary Kay came up for the family gathering instead. My relationship with my father would never be the same.

MY FRIEND LAURIE DIDN'T believe me when I told her that I'd never been to a therapist.

Shut up, she said. *How is that even possible?*

It just is, I said. I felt that I was getting the emotional support I needed from my family and friends. I had my coping strategies and ways to escape. I prayed first thing each day, walked to the lake each morning, did yoga, gardened, rode my bike, listened to Cubs games, drank beer, watched goofy shows, and read good books.

Still.

You gotta go see someone, she said.

She was right. I'd been so rattled after our family photos ended up in boxes at the rummage sale and Holmer's wife's ugly accusations that I was quick to tears, angry, and confused. All that unresolved trauma was catching up to me. The irony was not lost on me that I had been so busy writing newspaper stories about people needing better access to mental health care that I was neglecting my own.

The truth is, I was scared. I'd always fancied myself as the Marilyn Munster of the family, the normal one. But, deep down inside, I knew that wasn't really true. I also needed help.

Laurie gave me the name of her therapist. Her office was on the floor above a bank about three miles from our house—close enough that I worried someone might see me in the waiting room. In fact, when I walked in, I spotted a guy I worked with at the newspaper, one of my role models, sitting near the receptionist, his nose buried in a *New Yorker.* We both pretended not to see one another.

When the therapist called me into her office, she lit a candle and some incense. *Classic,* I thought. But I'd also imagined she'd have me lie on a couch while she faced away from me, scribbling notes, like they do in the movies. Instead, she had me sit across from her. *Tell me about your family,* she said. I swallowed hard.

How many days do you have?

As I started in, talking first about Nancy, then my mother, then Holmer and Danny, her eyes got bigger and bigger. I got the feeling she was trying not to gasp, and I imagined her reaching under her desk to push a button and the doors would swing open. Two brawny men in white coats would come with a straitjacket to take me away.

Then, I got to the story about the baby pictures and the suggestion that I had inappropriate feelings toward my father, and I could feel my cheeks start to flush. *I think you'd do well with some psychoanalysis,* the therapist said when our time expired. *When can you come back?*

Come back? One session had been more than enough. I could not imagine anything scarier or painfuller than slow walking through the events of my life and analyzing them for meaning. Nope. I was not ready for that, thank you very much.

Let me go home and look at my calendar, and I'll call you back so we can set up some time, I lied.

I never saw her again.

JAKE UNDERSTOOD WHY HE'D need to move from the condo, and he took the news with his signature grace. He said he was luckier than most, getting to live rent-free for so long in a pretty place just blocks from his beloved Lake Michigan. It would be impossible to find a place like that, or any place in the neighborhood that he could afford. Rents on Chicago's North Shore were among the highest in the country.

Mary Kay offered to help him find a place, one they both hoped wouldn't make him feel too lonely. Jake loved the jazz of our big family and remembered how depressed he'd been living alone in college. His best bet was a transitional group home about three miles away run by the nonprofit mental health agency that had helped Nancy decades earlier. But he couldn't just sign up and get a room. As I learned through my reporting, available housing for people with persistent mental illness is scarce. The wait can be more than a year. Often the places are run-down, and some are downright dangerous.

The place Mary Kay found with the help of Jake's caseworker was convenient, near enough that Jake could get to the lake and visit regularly with his girlfriend. There was a hitch: The place was established for people who are homeless. If he was going to qualify for a spot there, he'd have to scam his way in. Iconoclast that he is—ever eager to stick it to the Man—Jake jumped at the challenge.

The surest bet to establish Jake as homeless was for him to show up at a shelter for two nights in a row and get a card signed by the staff. Mary Kay was nervous about the safety of the place and made Jake promise to check in with her regularly by text. Jake, who'd apprenticed as a plumber years earlier, kept himself busy throughout the nights by fixing the shelter's toilets. Except for getting a parking ticket on the first night, his scheme worked well. Jake got approval to move into the group home the following week.

Holmer, who once petitioned to keep a group home out of our neighborhood for fear of what it might do to property values, was now relieved that Jake had some place to live, transitional as it may be.

Holmer and his wife never did move out of the condo, nor did they ever go to visit Jake at his new place. A few of his wife's children chipped in and bought the condo, relieving them of all that debt. They let Holmer and his wife stay there for free. Their financial troubles, however, were far from over. Even after their reverse mortgage funds dried up, they kept traveling and buying fresh flowers, getting regular manicures and pedicures, and putting it all on one credit card after another. Their debts kept climbing.

INFORMED BY JAKE'S DILEMMA, I continued writing stories about the lousy housing options for people with severe mental illness in Milwaukee. I'd seen some of the hellholes where the subjects of my stories lived and wondered how it was that their case managers could put them in these dirty, often dangerous places. As I traveled around reporting, I'd noticed rat droppings, broken smoke alarms, missing windows, dangling electrical wires, broken toilets, and furnaces that failed to work, even in the dead of a Wisconsin winter. In one place, I saw a bloody razor blade on the floor while the residents roamed around in bare feet. Yes, it was good that most of these people weren't being warehoused in mental institutions far from town, but I wanted my readers to see that the alternative for many was just as dangerous and dehumanizing, maybe more so. We needed to do better.

To try to figure out the scope of this problem, I met with case managers at each agency that contracted with Milwaukee County to provide support services for people with serious mental illness. These are people who are too ill or confused to manage daily chores, like shopping for groceries or paying their bills. The managers I met were typically young, bighearted, overworked, and underpaid. For the most part, they were good people stuck in a bad system with few or no good options. Their job was to find housing for their clients, negotiate leases with landlords, make sure their clients got to the doctor, took their medication, and had enough to eat—jobs a family member might do. But so many family members had long since vanished, unable to handle the stress of dealing with their often-volatile relatives.

With my reporter's notebook in hand, I probed deeper, trying to get to the root of the problem. It wasn't enough for me to simply describe these god-awful living spaces. I wanted to put the finger on who was to blame. It wasn't the case managers. They were frustrated at having to send their clients to these disgusting places, but there were no alternatives. Many landlords wouldn't rent to people enrolled in community mental health care, fearing they'd trash their places—which, in fairness, sometimes happened. There were laws against this kind of discrimination, of course, but they were hard to document and even harder to enforce. Mostly, caseworkers looked the other way when their clients moved into these rat traps, figuring any housing was better than none at all.

At my request, the case managers gave me the addresses of some of the worst places they'd seen. From the list of more than two hundred addresses they mentioned, I ran building code inspection reports and cross-referenced them with the city's database of building code violations. Not surprisingly, I found thousands of violations that had not been enforced. Faulty wiring. Mold. Rats. Leaky roofs. Broken toilets. Building inspectors admitted to me that they'd seen dozens of these illegal group homes—"so many that we can't begin to count them all"—but they, too, looked the other way. Without too much effort, I'd discovered an underground network of stealth group homes and ersatz mental hospitals with many of the horrific conditions of those awful old state asylums but none of the oversight or accountability.

The city's building inspection manager told me that it was not unusual to find hungry tenants begging outside of the buildings where they lived because their landlords took their disability checks and did not leave them with enough to fill their stomachs.

Here were hundreds of the county's most vulnerable people living in dirty, dangerous hovels, ignored by city and county workers alike. One man had been dead in his bed for four days before the smell of his rotting corpse caused the building management to pry open the door. Another man fell to his death from his landlady's rotting wooden porch, giving her ample opportunity to steal his food stamps. I felt like a twenty-first-century Charles Dickens chronicling one atrocity after the next.

Of all the godforsaken buildings that I traipsed through over those months of our reporting—often with photographer Kris Wentz-Graf in tow—none was worse than the place where Bessie lived. We found Bessie lying on a urine-stained mattress with wads of spent toilet paper strewn around the room. The stench was so strong, I choked when I walked through the door. The landlady, who'd also spent time as a patient at the county mental health hospital, told me that she sometimes got food out of dumpsters that she would serve to the people who lived in her building.

"It's a lot cheaper that way," she told me.

She said county mental health managers got angry at her after two of her tenants died in one day, one from a heart attack and the other from heat exhaustion. People on psychiatric medications are especially vulnerable to heatstroke.

"What am I supposed to do?" the landlady said. "It's not my job to babysit these people." City building inspectors had cited her six times in three years for running illegal group homes, but she was never prosecuted. Still, county case managers kept contracting with her to place their clients in her houses. They'd come to the houses several times a week to check up on their clients, looking the other way at the bloody razor blade on the floor, the moldy eggs and expired cereal in the pantry, and the piles of used toilet paper stinking throughout the rooms. Most of their clients didn't seem to mind the filth either. They were so delusional and confused, they didn't know where they were.

Georgia Rawlings, a bawdy, foulmouthed, crack-smoking wisenheimer, was standing in the laundromat across the street, waving her cigarette, holding court when I met her.

"I said, 'No, fuck YOU!'" she shouted to no one in particular and then let out a roaring laugh. *My kind of woman,* I thought. I introduced myself and told her why I was there.

"Yeah, I used to live there," said Georgia, glancing across the street.

Tell me what it was like, I said. Georgia thought for a few seconds.

"Well, I might have bats in my belfry, but that lady has rats in her attic. Ha!"

I whipped out my notebook.

Georgia said she had lived in the house across the street a few years earlier but got kicked out for smoking crack. Ditto for the next place. Her caseworker had managed to set her up in a pretty good place for now, but the new landlady didn't want her smoking anything inside, not even cigarettes.

Georgia was fifty-four years old, with a round face and sparkling blue eyes. The few teeth she had were chipped and brown. She had a mischievous grin, tempting me to try to learn as much as I could about her. She talked like her mouth was full of marbles, most likely a side effect of the medication she took.

"I'm not from around here," she told me.

She said she grew up outside of Chicago, just north, in a town called Wilmette.

"Shut up!" I said, giving her a little push.

"No, YOU shut up," she said, pushing me right back.

Sure enough, Georgia and I had grown up about eight blocks from one another. She was the middle of five children. Her sisters called her "Wuggie." We joked about our shared Wilmette heritage—making out with boys in Gillson Park, tobogganing down Suicide Hill, ordering Green Rivers and plates of fries at Bob's Restaurant. Ann-Margret's old house was just a few blocks down from Georgia's and so was Bill Murray's.

"His sister, the nun, taught me drama in high school," I said.

We went on like this for quite a while, and that's when it hit me. Georgia was just a few years older than my sister Nancy.

"Hey, Georgia," I said. "Were you ever in Evanston Hospital in the early 1970s?"

Georgia leaned in and studied my face. She stepped in for closer inspection, and her eyes widened. Then she slapped her hand to her mouth.

"Kissinger. You and your sister Nancy have the same sad brown eyes," she whispered.

"Had," I said, amazed. "Nancy's dead now."

"Yeah," Georgia said. "I remember."

So, Georgia, Kris the photographer, and I took a little road trip down to Wilmette the next week. We had lunch with Georgia's two sisters and a niece who bummed a drag of Georgia's cigarette when her mother wasn't looking. "I'm contributing to the delinquency of a delinquent!" Georgia announced. After a quick tour of Gillson Park, we stopped in the alley behind the house where her sister Sandy had lived. Sandy, who was blind and had diabetes, had died a few months before Georgia and I met. The house was located just a few blocks from the train tracks where Nancy had been killed.

We sat there and talked about our sisters.

"God, I miss her," Georgia said of Sandy. She bowed her head and started to weep. *Me, too,* I said, thinking of Nancy.

For the next several years, Georgia became a kind of tour guide for me as I navigated the world of substandard housing for people with severe mental illness. I watched as she got kicked out of her new place for smoking and then the next one and the next. She ultimately ended up in a trailer park near Milwaukee's airport that was later profiled in Matthew Desmond's Pulitzer Prize–winning book, *Evicted: Poverty and Profit in the American City.*

In time, Georgia became more of a friend than a source. I stopped writing about her, not wanting to compromise our relationship, and took my kids to the trailer park each Christmas Eve for a little gift exchange.

"Honey, kid," she said when I walked in the trailer with a bag of Burger King hamburgers and some fries one Christmas Eve.

"Ho, ho, ho," I said, handing her the food.

She grabbed the bag and frowned. "Who you callin' a ho?"

If I closed my eyes, I could pretend that Georgia was Nancy. They both loved blowing smoke rings and bragging about how much trouble they could cause. Georgia had a stroke in the spring of 2011. I went to the ICU and held her hand, grateful for the chance to offer her the tenderness I had never been able to share with Nancy.

Georgia rallied but died the next May. She was sixty-two. I was honored when her sisters called and asked me to go back to Wilmette to give her eulogy.

"It's not always easy to look past the label of someone's illness to see the person they are inside," I told the crowd in church that afternoon. "If you could do that with Georgia, you were in for a treat. She was one of the smartest, funniest, and most generous people around. I loved her."

The same could have been said about Nancy. I just didn't have the chance.

My stories had gained traction. Two days after the first story ran, the director of the county's mental health division was fired for allowing his case managers to put their clients in unsafe, illegal group homes. Federal housing managers called out city bureaucrats who failed to go after millions of dollars of available funding for housing projects like the kind Jake was now living in, ones Milwaukee dearly needed.

My editors were urging me to grill politicians and bureaucrats about why they were abandoning the people who needed them most. They ran my stories at the top of page 1 in hopes that we could shame officials into action. To our delight, the politicians took the bait we lobbed day after day from our bully pulpit.

Tom Barrett, the Democratic mayor, and county executive Scott Walker, a Republican, set aside their political differences and announced a host of reforms, including a new hybrid department of housing for people with mental illness. Eventually, more than one thousand new units of clean, affordable supportive housing would be built.

As gratifying as that was, I had no time for a victory lap. My inbox was full of desperate pleas for help from people wanting me to call attention to the poor care that their family members were getting. Jean Anczak's daughter, Cindy, lost twenty-two pounds in three weeks as a patient at the county-run psychiatric hospital before dying of complications from malnutrition and dehydration. "What kind of hospital lets you starve to death?" she asked. "We treat animals better than this."

Each day, it seemed, I was learning of one more outrage after another, some vulnerable person with severe mental illness whose case had been badly botched or they couldn't get any help at all.

Larry was traveling a lot for business, and Charley and Molly were now away at college. I'd come home late at night, crack open a cold beer, and stare into space. Then I'd leaf through the day's mail. One evening, I found a letter from my doctor's office, saying the mammogram they'd taken a week earlier had been inconclusive. I'd need to go back and have more images taken.

Oh, shit, I thought, trying not to overreact. A good friend's wife had been diagnosed with breast cancer. *It's ninety-nine point nine percent likely nothing,* I told myself. *People redo these mammograms all the time.*

Still more annoyed than worried, I went in a few days later for a follow-up mammogram and planned to meet my friends Laurie and Katie for lunch afterward.

Just a few more, Margaret, the radiation technician said. I waited on the table while they took another look. She returned.

Guess we might need a few more pictures, she said with a nervous laugh as she sent me back for a third round. *Did she look worried?* I wondered. *This doesn't seem normal. Am I being dramatic?*

I checked my watch. Laurie and Katie would be waiting.

15 more minutes, I texted them.

Nancy the nurse came back into the room.

We're gonna need to do a biopsy, she said. She wasn't smiling anymore.

Now I was scared.

Go ahead without me, I texted my friends. Apparently, I might have cancer.

Laurie texted back immediately: !!!!!!!!!!!!!!!!!

A while later, Nancy the nurse came in with the doctor and took hold of my hand.

We're pretty sure it's cancer, the doctor said. *But we won't know for sure until the pathology report comes back tomorrow.*

Margaret, Nancy said, double-checking my chart to be sure she'd called me by the right name. *This will give you character.*

After all that our family had been through, I didn't think I needed any more character.

But I have too much already, I said as I started to cry. *I have too much fucking character.*

Nancy tucked a booklet under my arm, titled "Understanding Breast Cancer."

Whatever you do, don't go on the internet, she said. *It'll just scare you.*

So, I went home and went on the internet.

It scared me.

I knew almost nothing about breast cancer, except that it had killed my grandmother when she was the same age that I was. I did not want it to kill me. Unlike Nancy and Danny and others in my family, I'd never considered suicide. In fact, I very much wanted to stay alive at all costs.

I'd just written a series for the newspaper on a radiation oncologist who diagnosed his own stage IV esophageal cancer and watched as he struggled to come to terms with the illness that would soon kill him. Now months of chemotherapy and radiation for me? *I don't have time for cancer right now,* I told the doctor when he called the next day to confirm my biopsy results. I see now that I must have been a bit shell-shocked to realize how ridiculous that sounded.

Then the gravity of my situation started to sink in. *Oh my God. Am I going to die now?* Our daughter, Molly, had just started college at the University of Wisconsin, and Charley was in his junior year at Northwestern (yeah, HE got in). There was still so much I wanted to help them navigate—fussy roommates, broken hearts, choosing a career, falling in love, graduations, weddings, babies. I couldn't bear the thought of leaving them or Larry. Besides, I was on the journalistic roll of my life, doing what Danny had challenged me to do—putting human faces on mental illness and daring people to look away. My stories about Georgia and John Spoerl and dozens of others were prompting real, sustained change that would help people live better lives.

Now I'd have to find a way to keep my own life going.

15
Holmer in the Gloamin'

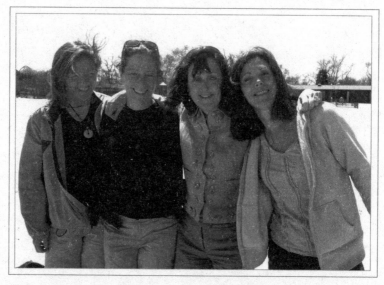

Holmer's "semi-beautiful daughters" at the Wilmette beach.
Left to right: Molly, Patty, me, and Mary Kay.
(Photo credit: Molly Boynton)

Larry came into the upstairs study where I'd been lying on the couch, looking at the moon shining over Lake Michigan. It was somewhere around 2:30 in the morning, and the February wind was howling.

What are you doing in here? he said, kneeling at my side.

I'm bald, and my mouth hurts, I said. *I can't sleep.*

My hair had fallen out a few days earlier after the second round of chemotherapy, and my mouth was full of sores. I had two more rounds of chemo to go followed by thirty-seven radiation treatments. I never considered myself to be vain, so I was surprised by how rattled I was when my hair fell out. And cold. I bought a wig, but I hated it. It reminded me of the terrible, ill-fitting one that my mother used to wear just before she died. Her "hair helmet," as Holmer called it, made her look like a skeleton. So, we put my wig on our beagle and on our funny neighbor Dan from across the street.

I'm not mature enough to be a good cancer patient, I told my kids.

Lying there alone in the middle of the night, I felt ugly and scared and very sorry for myself. The odds were in my favor, but, in my overly dramatic brain, getting cancer means you will die from it, probably sooner than later. *Gee,* Larry said, taking my hand as I started to cry. *Next time you can't sleep, wake me. I'll stay up with you.*

I couldn't imagine a more perfect thing for him to say.

Chemo had taken its toll on me. I was tired and even more easily distracted than normal, which I didn't think was possible. I couldn't multitask anymore and had a hard time remembering much. So, it was a relief when George Stanley, then the managing editor at the *Milwaukee Journal Sentinel,* assigned me to work alongside Susanne Rust, a young science writer without much daily newspaper experience but lots of savvy and a killer instinct for news. We were to examine the debate around the safety of bisphenol A, or BPA, a chemical used to make thousands of household products, including baby bottles. A growing legion of scientists worried that the chemical, suspected of causing cancer and other maladies in lab animals, might do the same to humans. The only health reporting I'd done concerned mental health, but many of the themes were the same. We'd be investigating why the government was not doing more to protect vulnerable people.

Susanne and I made quite a team. For the next three years, we dug into the secret alliances between government regulators and chemical manufacturers. Our stories revealed how entire sections of the government's safety assessments were being ghostwritten by the companies that made the chemicals. Even with my limited knowledge of science, I knew that was akin to having the proverbial fox guard the henhouse. Our stories drew national attention and enough journalism award plaques to fill both of our office walls. We were named as finalists for the Pulitzer Prize in investigative reporting.

Working with Susanne, I learned how to go for the jugular, to dig for evidence of wrongdoing, showing how people with power manipulate the system. It wasn't enough to just tell sad stories of people who'd been injured in some way. You had to follow the money, reveal conflicts of interest, expose the culprits, and hold them to account.

SOMETIMES THE BAD GUYS are too close for comfort. Jake called me at the newsroom in a panic one spring day. He said Holmer and his wife were using his credit card, and Jake was afraid of what would happen if they ran up the balance so high that he wouldn't be able to pay it off. Unlike Holmer, Jake had an excellent credit score.

What the hell are you talking about? I asked Jake. Could it really be possible that Holmer and his wife were now grifting Jake? They had just declared bankruptcy and had no way to get credit on their own. Once they had spent all the equity from the condominium—more than $300,000— they racked up another $164,000 in credit card charges. According to the bankruptcy filings, they maxed out three separate Macy's credit cards, four Chase cards, three for Capital One, two Citibank cards, and a host of other cards, including Bloomingdale's, Lord & Taylor, Saks Fifth Avenue, and Neiman Marcus. And now it seemed they were moving on to Jake's.

What if he needs the money for chemo? Jake said, near tears. *I want to help him.*

He doesn't need your money, I assured Jake. Holmer had recently been diagnosed with melanoma. The cancer was slow growing, the doctor said, but there would be no cure. Holmer had Medicare and Veterans Administration benefits from his eighteen months in the navy during World War II. Just to be sure, I had Jake check to see what they were using his card for. It was just as I feared: gourmet popcorn, tires for Holmer's car, and some goddamn fresh flowers delivered to their house.

Lower your card limit to a thousand dollars ASAP, I told him. There was no telling how much more cheesy wall art or jewelry these people could rack up in short order. That way, in the worst-case scenario, Jake would be on the hook for only $1,000, a sum I knew he had in his bank account.

What the hell, Holmer? I barked at my father when I called him a few minutes later. *Now you're putting the squeeze on Jake? Jake who lives in a group home for homeless people and can't work because of his crippling depression and anxiety? You're creating MORE anxiety for him?* I understood that Holmer's bipolar illness made him do some crazy shit, but this was about the lowest thing I could imagine. I was furious.

This is none of your goddamn business, Holmer told me and hung up.

So I sent an email to all my siblings and Holmer's wife's children, telling them what had happened and how unacceptable this was. *We need a game plan,* I said. *Clearly, these people do not know how to manage their money. What if we came up with a budget for them and between all of us kids, we could cover whatever else they needed. Who's in?*

A few of my siblings were on board, but I never heard back from any of Holmer's wife's children. Three weeks later, Holmer and his wife paid Jake back the money they owed him.

BY 2009, SUSANNE WAS off to California for a Knight Foundation journalism fellowship, and I was back to full health. Or at least as "full health" as I'd ever allow myself to imagine. By then, I'd been to enough funerals for friends who thought they were in remission from breast cancer to know better than to consider myself "cured." Denice Stingl, the wife of one of my best newsroom buddies, was diagnosed five years before I was with a nearly identical profile and prognosis. She brought me meals, cheered me up, and warned me that the chemo might kill the feeling in my fingers and toes. Radiation, she told me, will burn my skin to blisters. When her cancer came roaring back eleven years after she was declared "free and clear," I knew I would never stop looking over my shoulder.

My friend Ann asked me to help her write goodbye letters to her two teenage kids after her cancer came back, but the disease spread so fast, there wasn't time. I'd always felt badly that they didn't have those words on paper from their mother letting them know how she felt. Knowing that whatever cancer cells might be hiding in my body could start multiplying like crazy at any minute, I felt an added urgency now to do the things I needed to get done. I was itching to get back to stories about our country's lousy mental health system. There was no shortage of outrages to report. But the stories that astounded me the most were the cover-ups of abuses by those who were trusted to help.

A FEDERAL INSPECTION REPORT issued in March 2010 declared patients at the Milwaukee County Mental Health Complex to be in immediate jeopardy after a rash of sexual assaults against female patients there. Four women were reported to have been attacked by the same man, including one woman with severe developmental disabilities who had become pregnant. The man, twenty-two, had a history of violence and sexual assault, but was still permitted to come and go from the hospital as he wished. He'd once punched a nurse with such force that he broke the man's eye socket. Steve Schultze, the newspaper's county government reporter, and I spent the next several months investigating the hospital.

By 2010, almost 90 percent of the hospital beds across the country that were once available for the sickest psychiatric patients had been eliminated. Those who were committed to long-term care were sicker and more violent than patients in the past. Hospital administrators had trouble hiring and retaining good doctors and nurses. The doctor in charge of the pregnant woman's care had his license suspended for two years in 1987 after admitting to having sex regularly with two of his patients. The same doctor had supervised Cindy Anczak, the woman who died in 2006 of complications from starvation and dehydration.

The pregnant woman's guardian had asked that the patient be put on birth control injections when she was admitted the previous July, but for some reason the hospital staff did not do that. The guardian was furious about how the hospital had botched her client's case. The attack happened that same day that the woman was admitted, but she was not given a pregnancy test for nearly two months. Even then, the guardian was not told of the pregnancy for several more weeks, so abortion was no longer an option. All the while, hospital staff continued to give the woman three highly potent antipsychotics a day, medication that might have harmed her developing fetus.

State inspection reports we got through open records requests showed that nursing assistants and administrators mismanaged the case from the beginning, ignored medical orders, and falsified documents to hide their mistakes.

Readers were outraged. The hospital director appeared before the county board, which oversaw operations at the public facility, to explain why this was happening. The director said he and his staff consciously decided to house men and women on the same ward, even knowing the risks to the female patients. Sexual assaults in mixed-gender wards, he said, were a "trade-off" for more violent assaults that would happen in all-male psychiatric units. The idea of a sexual assault as an acceptable trade-off was too much for people to bear. The director was fired the day after our story appeared.

Scott Walker, the county executive, was running for governor of Wisconsin and did not want a scandal like this to taint his record and ruin his chances at election. His minions were scrambling to contain the damage.

"Last week was a nightmare," wrote Kelly Rindfleisch, Walker's deputy chief of staff, in emails we later obtained through an open records request. "A bad story every day on our looney bin. Doctors having sex with patients, patients getting knocked up. This has been coming for months and I've unofficially been dealing with it. So, it's been crazy (pun intended)."

Despite this, Rindfleisch wrote in a later email, she believed Walker would prevail in his election bid. The cause for her optimism was as cynical as it was cruel: "No one cares about crazy people." But it was also correct, apparently.

Three months later, Walker won the gubernatorial election, handily.

AFTER YEARS OF STAYING at bay, Holmer's cancer was now spreading to his lungs and brain. I started to visit him regularly again, awkward as it was. He was my father, and I loved him, and I knew he loved me. Still, his wife always made sure to stay in the room.

My siblings were also checking in on Holmer often now, treating him to flourishes we knew he could no longer afford—a subscription to a music streaming service so he could listen to his beloved jazz, a new washer and dryer, special pillows, even a hydraulic lift chair to get him up and down the stairs, a contraption that Mary Kay called *Disney for old people.* Yes, it was his own damn fault that he'd blown all his money—and then some—and was now unable to buy these things for himself. But we also knew that he'd sacrificed plenty for us over the years, and no one wanted to deny him a comfortable last few months, or however much time he had left.

YOUR FATHER WOULD LIKE *to see you,* Holmer's wife said when she called me on a Friday morning in April 2011. *The doctors think it won't be much longer.*

By the time I got to the hospital ninety minutes later, Billy, Mary Kay, and Jake were in the hallway, cracking little jokes, waiting for me so we could all go in together.

Sounds like my Zumba class in here, Mary Kay said as classical Latin music thumped quietly through the speaker system.

We'd gathered in this very hospital many times before, but under much different circumstances. Nancy's death, declared in the emergency room downstairs thirty-three years earlier, had been so sudden, we had no chance to say goodbye. Our mother died just down the hall from where we were standing. Her death had been gentle and peaceful, but she had just started coming into her own. We hadn't been ready to lose her. And then there was Danny, of course. Holmer, by contrast, had had a good, long run. He was eighty-four. So, when his wife called to summon us all, I felt like we'd been given a gift, the chance to say goodbye to someone who'd lived a long, full life.

She cracked open the door and then left us alone with him for a change. One by one, we tiptoed into the room and formed a kind of human shroud around our father's bed. The curtains were drawn. Not that it mattered on such a gray April day, but the darkness made it difficult for us to see him. So, we huddled at his side, our shoulders touching, the way they did on hot summer nights when we were small. We'd line up our sleeping bags on our parents' air-conditioned bedroom floor and snuggle in tight. *Shush up!!* we'd whisper to each other as we lay in the dark, fearing too much noise would wake Holmer and he'd start swinging away. So we'd swallow hard, fighting back the urge to giggle by biting our pillows so hard that we could feel the spines of the feathers crunch.

Now, all these years later, we stood before the old tiger, who was curled up like a helpless kitten. No more jabbing elbows or punching fists. No more teeth.

I reached for Holmer's hand, relieved at how warm it felt.

A Holmer in the gloamin', I leaned over and whispered to Billy, referencing one of the most famous home runs in baseball history.

As Holmer lay dying in the hospice room, it was strange to see him, the charmer who could talk his way in or out of almost anything, unable to speak. Just a week earlier, we'd been goofing around in his hospital room, watching the Cubs blow a three-run lead on the TV.

How much for that? Holmer whispered, pointing to my new iPad. *I want one.*

This guy and his bells and whistles, I thought. *Still trying to work a grift.*

You won't be needing this where you're going, old man, I told him. *It's all one big iPad up there.*

Since Holmer arrived at the hospice in early April, his room had been the scene of a steady parade of fans and old friends. His former fiancée, my mother's dear pal, stopped by one day. They held hands for a bit and recalled old times. *See you on the other side,* Holmer whispered as she headed toward the door. The next day, a friend of his wife's came to sing some church hymns. Holmer listened earnestly, his eyes closed and his hands crossed reverently over his chest, but the second she ducked out to use the bathroom, Holmer motioned for me to come to his side.

Get that broad outta here, he whispered in my ear. *She's driving me out of my fucking mind.*

Holmer stopped talking two days later and could only suck on ice chips. *Not too much longer now,* the nurse said. We called the hospital each morning to see how he was doing, but his wife had instructed the nurses' station not to give out reports of his condition to anyone but her.

So, now, here we were, back at the hospital again, probably for the last time, fidgeting, wondering what to do. No one was ready to say goodbye.

We fumbled for our phones, trying to get Patty on the line from New Orleans and Molly, who was teaching kiteboarding somewhere in the Baja.

We tucked one cell phone under each of his arms and made time for a few little stories: *Remember the night he marched us up the side of the mountain in Steamboat Springs so we could count the falling stars?* Jake asked.

He cried at how beautiful they were, Billy said.

Patty's turn: *He took me—and ONLY me—to see Woody Herman play at Old Orchard one summer night.*

Molly recalled how Holmer coached her grade school basketball team and the girls made a big thank-you card for him that read THE COACH IS NO ROACH!!!! A few years later, Holmer, now a mere spectator, made so much commotion from the stands after what he considered to be a bad call that the ref imposed a technical foul on Molly's team and they lost the game.

It was time to let Holmer rest, but no one wanted to leave just yet.

We kept stalling but we couldn't stand next to his bed forever.

Hey, shouldn't we say a rosary or something? I asked. No answer. So, I asked again. It seemed like the right thing to do.

The rituals of our Catholic upbringing comfort me. But most of my siblings had soured on the church years earlier, disgusted at bishops' handling of the sexual abuse scandal, the disregard for women's rights and equality, and its labeling of LGBTQ+ people as "disordered." I shared their disapproval on all of these matters—but chose to stay and fight for reforms from within. Was I wimping out?

This was neither the time nor the place for such debate. I respected their choices and hoped they respected mine. Still, I thought it would comfort Holmer to have us recite something familiar in solidarity, a kind of team cheer. Any old communal verse would do. A few weeks earlier, Charley and

I had sat on either side of Holmer as he lay in bed, holding his hands while we sang church songs. *I will go, Lord, if you lead me.*

Nice lyrics. Wrong crowd. Plan B:

How about "Walla Walla, Washington"?

This was our favorite family song, the one we sang on car trips to Wisconsin and out to Colorado, the ten of us smushed into one station wagon. Holmer, one hand on the wheel, the other scratching his scalp. My mother would sing along with a kid or two on her lap. The rest of us would join in from the middle seat or the very back section of our station wagon.

Walla Walla, Washington. I started and they all followed. *Walla Walla, Washington.* Before long, we were on a roll.

Walla Walla, Walla Walla, Walla Walla, Walla Walla, Washington.

I wondered what the other families down the hall at the hospice were thinking as we warbled on.

This would be the perfect time for the old coot to give up the ghost, I thought.

But nobody puts Holmie in the corner. He lived by his own rules, and he would die by them, too. Good Friday was just a week away, the day that Christians commemorate the crucifixion and death of Christ. We were pretty sure he was holding out for that day so that we would all make the comparison.

We always assumed that Holmer would be buried next to our mother. Holmer used to joke that, should he ever remarry, *put me between my two wives, but roll me over a little closer to your mother.*

But his new wife did not want to be buried up in Milwaukee. A few weeks earlier, we had dispatched Billy to try to figure out what we should do. He went over to the condo one afternoon while Holmer was still at home. Though weak, Holmer was still lucid and able to talk. Billy asked him what his wishes were. *I want to be buried next to your mother,* he said.

Billy pressed him. *You sure about that?*

Holmer said he was.

Since we knew neither Holmer nor his wife had the money to pay for a funeral, some of my siblings and I decided that we would pitch in and give him the kind of send-off he'd always said he wanted: a nice long wake, followed the next day by a funeral mass and then a lunch for all the mourners, maybe not at the preferred Michigan Shores Club, but some place nice enough, where we could hoist a Bloody Mary or a glass of chardonnay and tell all the stories about him that were too saucy to recite in a church.

Holmer's wife was in the kitchen when Billy came downstairs to tell her what had been decided. Her face fell. *Oh, no,* she said. *That is not what we talked about at all.* She said that they had decided to be cremated and have their ashes buried together. Billy shrugged, unsure of how to reconcile these vastly different plans. The two of them marched back upstairs, hoping for clarity. Holmer's eyes darted back and forth. He wasn't up for a fight. *I don't give a shit what you do with me,* he said. *Burn me up for all I care and split the ashes in two.*

Oh, the wisdom of Solomon, his wife said with a smile.

So, that's what we did. Holmer died on Holy Thursday, six hours short of his presumed timeline.

It was real gentle, Jake said when he called to give me the news as I was driving down to be with them. Hard to imagine. That might have been the only time I heard the word *gentle* used to describe anything about my father.

The next week, Mary Kay picked up Holmer's ashes from the discount crematorium. As planned, she poured some in a jar for his wife and some in another jar to be buried next to our mother. Never one to abide protocol, Mary Kay saved a few teaspoons for herself, which she scooped into an I Can't Believe It's Not Butter! container, to be scattered later at a date and place of her choosing.

Billy delivered the eulogy to a standing-room-only crowd, nailing a perfect imitation of Holmer moving some porch furniture—*LOOK OUT NOW, I'M COMIN' OUT SWINGIN!'* Billy recalled how Holmer referred to Mary Kay, Patty, Molly and me as his "semi-beautiful daughters," and how he wanted his tombstone to read SEE, I TOLD YOU I WAS SICK. If you were walking by the church that morning, you might have thought it was open mic at a comedy club. I still get requests for copies.

Holmer's wife said she didn't have the energy to come up to Milwaukee the following Monday for the ceremony to bury our half of his ashes. So, I arranged for an honor guard to give a twenty-one-gun salute, and they presented the flag to Mary Kay. The pomp may have been a bit disproportionate to Holmer's valor during his brief stint in stateside duty at the tail end of World War II, but, considering how the military had screwed his parents when Uncle Jack was killed, we figured it was the least they could do. Then we all went back to my house, played a few games of Wiffle ball, and ate takeout Chinese food. After dinner, our bellies full of MSG and IPAs, we spread out on the family room floor and fought to stay awake watching *Best in Show*.

With both of our parents now dead, my siblings and I knew that we would need to make an extra effort to stay connected. The rest of us had jobs and our own families to keep us busy, but Jake was on his own now. We worried about what might happen if he began feeling sad and lonely.

It didn't take long for us to find out.

16

Be Wounded by
the Stories You Tell

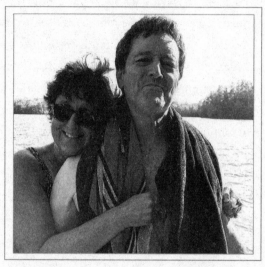

*Jake and me, back on the pier where Jake rescued me
after I'd fallen in so many years earlier, in Land O' Lakes,
Wisconsin, 2021. (Photo credit: Shelly Weingarten)*

Jake's caseworker sent me an email just after Christmas that year to let me know that my brother was struggling. "He said he'd like to live with family again until he feels better," she wrote. "He specifically mentioned you."

My first instinct was to jump at the chance to invite Jake to move in with Larry and me. "No threepeats," we all vowed at Danny's funeral. We'd learned the hard way what could happen if you turned away from someone having a "hard molt." Besides, Jake was easier to deal with than

Nancy and Danny. He was not too proud to say that he was struggling and to ask one of us for help. I was flattered that he thought of me.

Larry and I had been empty nesters for a few years by then, so our house was big enough to accommodate him. I imagined Jake helping Larry in his vegetable garden and the three of us going on great weekend adventures—long bike rides on the Elroy-Sparta State Trail, canoeing the mighty Kickapoo River, or hiking in the Kettle Moraine State Forest. *It'll be fun,* I told Larry. Milwaukee, less than two hours from Chicago, is famous for its gemütlichkeit, with lots of craft breweries, great music festivals, and plenty of action along the shores of Jake's beloved Lake Michigan.

But, of course, there were more complicating factors to consider.

Jake is a bit of a mad scientist. He makes homemade wine out of what many people would consider garbage. One sweltering August day, he tried to thaw some frozen chicken on the hood of his car. More than once, the fire department had been called to his group home after Jake's plan to make candles out of animal fat went awry.

He can also be fussy about the thermostat. Because the medication he takes inhibits his ability to sweat, Jake wilts in the heat. He likes the air conditioner to be turned on any time the temperature gets above seventy-five degrees. We prefer open windows and fresh air from nearby Lake Michigan. Whereas Larry and I are early birds, Jake tends to be a night owl, particularly when he's having trouble sleeping. Other times, he hops in and out of bed most of the day and putters around the house. He'd miss his social life. Jake's longtime girlfriend, Annie, lived in Wilmette with her parents. Jake's doctors were in Chicago. I worried about whether Milwaukee would be too socially isolating for him. And what about his disability benefits? Would they transfer from one state to the next?

Let's just take our time and think this through, Larry said.

Still, I was nervous. Did we have time to think this through? Jake hadn't been suicidal since he was hospitalized just before Holmer's wedding twelve years earlier. But no one wanted to take a chance that he might start to feel that way again. I was acutely aware of how deadly mental illness can be, even more so of late.

Just a few months earlier, I was the one who had tipped off the police that Jim Hankin was probably dead.

JIM AND I HAD what he called a "mental relationship." We both got a kick out of that double meaning. Our relationship began sometime in 1992 when he called me at the newsroom to warn me that a conservative radio talk show host was talking some smack on me for the little gossip column I was writing at the time. People used to call the newsroom all the time to talk about the craziest things. To me, that was one of the perks of the job. Jim reminded me a bit of Jake—bright, thoughtful, quirky, and vulnerable.

I never knew what his actual psychiatric diagnosis was. But, if I had to guess, I'd say Jim was on the autism spectrum with obsessive-compulsive disorder and ever-intensifying fear of leaving home.

Jim was in his early forties the first time he called me. He was caring for his father, a retired lawyer and bar association president, who had suffered a stroke. I could tell that Jim was a little off. But I was touched by his devotion to his parents. My mother had just died, and I was wistful. I let that slip into the conversation, and I think Jim saw that as an invitation to try to help me, too. From that day on, he'd call every now and then to see how I was doing.

Sometimes, he held up the phone so that he and his father could sing a song or tell me a joke. Usually, we'd talk for just a minute or two. Other times, we'd chat for an hour, mostly about politics but sometimes about family.

Before I knew it, Jim was bringing me baskets of blackberries from the bushes in his backyard. Larry and I took Charley and Molly to his house for trick-or-treating on Halloween. When Jim's father died, I went to the funeral, and that kind of locked me into Jim's good graces.

"You're a chronic sweetheart," he told me.

I wasn't. Sometimes, I was too busy to take his calls. Other times, I just wasn't in the mood. I'd let the phone ring, thankful for Caller ID.

The five hundred or more voice mails he left for me over the years always started like this:

"Well, it's [fill in the precise time] here in wonderful Whitefish Bay, Wisconsin. Hi, Meg. It's Jim, of course."

After his mother died, Jim was on his own. The paint on the shutters blistered, and the weeds began to sprout from the cracks on the sidewalk in front of his house. Neighbors called the village clerk to complain. Mothers warned their kids not to play in his yard or eat the blackberries from the bushes. His house was crammed with so many old tin cans and piles of newspaper that even a cat would have a hard time slinking into some of the rooms.

But I knew that Jim, like Boo Radley from *To Kill a Mockingbird*, was more complicated than people gave him credit for. Our conversations grew more serious. He hinted at having been institutionalized in high school. He filled in some details about his illness, but not many.

"We'll talk about that some other time," he'd say.

Frankly, I wasn't sure I wanted to know more. I just saw Jim as a lonely guy who needed a little conversation with the outside world.

Jim started becoming more reclusive. He stopped driving his car and started getting his groceries and medications delivered. One day in mid-July 2011, he called to say he was having health issues, and he wondered if I could drive him to the doctor. The appointment was set for 1:30 p.m. on August 4. Reluctantly, I agreed. Holmer had just died, and the story I was working on was emotionally draining. As selfish as this may sound, I wasn't sure I had the bandwidth to deal with Jim. I wonder now if Jim sensed my hesitation. He called the day before the appointment to say he was not well enough to go. No amount of coaxing could get him to see that was exactly why he needed to go. He rescheduled for August 24.

"Can I bring you some soup?" I asked, feeling a little guilty for balking at his earlier request.

Jim demurred. "Maybe next week when my tummy feels better," he said.

This was a stickier situation than I wanted to be in. I understood that Jim wanted his privacy and independence, but I also felt that if he was as sick as he seemed to be, I, or someone in his family, had an obligation to get him help. I called his cousin in St. Louis, who promised to call Jim. I vowed to check on Jim every few days. When I didn't hear from him the following Saturday, I hopped on my bike and pedaled to his house.

No answer. Neither of the next-door neighbors was home. So, I left a message with the woman in the house to the north, whom I had met a few times over the years. She called two days later to say that Jim had not put out the trash that morning. More alarmingly, he'd not called to wish her son a happy birthday, something he did religiously to many of his friends and neighbors. She and I knew that Jim would never skip a birthday call unless something was terribly wrong.

My heart pounding, I called the police.

When I got to Jim's house, they were trying to figure out a way to get in without breaking down the door. When that proved impossible, they used a crowbar.

The neighbors and I stood in Jim's backyard, straining to recall the last time any of us had seen him face-to-face. It had been years. After about twenty minutes, a young cop came out to confirm what we all feared. They found Jim facedown in the hallway, clutching his stomach. The police figured that he had been dead for four or five days. An autopsy would later show that Jim died of complications from a bladder infection that four dollars' worth of antibiotics could have cleared up in a few days.

It was 10:08 a.m. in wonderful Whitefish Bay, Wisconsin. And Jim Hankin's body was being loaded onto the coroner's stretcher.

Like so many people with mental illness, Jim died alone. What part had I played in that? Had Jim canceled his doctor's appointment because he sensed that I didn't want to leave work to drive him?

We are NOT going to let that happen to Jake, I thought.

LARRY AND I HAD been planning a trip to Mexico with Jake that February to visit our sister Molly and her three little children in the Baja. Molly had moved out west in the late 1980s, a few years after college, forsaking her promising career as a marketing manager in Philadelphia and New York City for a life of skiing, snowboarding, kiteboarding, and yoga. She and her partner and their kids lived off the grid, toggling their time between a yurt on the beach in the Baja and a barn in the mountains of Hood River, Oregon. This visit with them would be a perfect opportunity to see if Larry, Jake, and I could live together long-term without driving each other nuts. We pitched our tents on the beach in the shadow of Molly's yurt, and our little dress rehearsal was underway.

Our week in Mexico whizzed by. One day, we went to the Pacific side of the peninsula and watched gray whales spout. Another day, we walked the beaches south of La Paz and bobbed in the turquoise water as pelicans flew overhead. We scuba dived with dolphins, drank Dos Equis, and played Hearts, a favorite card game from our old ski trip days. *Smoke 'er out, smoke 'er out, smoke 'er out, out, OUT,* we chanted, remembering the song Holmer always sang in search of the dangerous queen of spades.

It was sweet to say good night to each other, knowing we would wake up the next day and play the way we had when we were kids.

Just before dinner on the evening before we left, some sea turtles laid their eggs on the beach, and this created a great commotion. These animals are precious, and the people of La Ventana go to great lengths to protect them. By the time we got to the shore, a crowd had gathered, cameras clicking, people bending forward, stretching their necks for a better view down the deep black hole.

"Apuro! Hurry!" a young boy said to his mother as she scooped the eggs from the hole and gently placed them into a Styrofoam box. Later, she would bury the eggs in a nest away from the water where kiteboarders and windsurfers could not smash them.

The Mexican sky glowed hot pink as the sun started to set. I stood there next to Jake and thought about how the same kind of drama was playing out between us.

Life and death and the urgent need to keep each other safe. We help protect one another because we are family, and that's what good families do.

By the time we got home, Jake said he was feeling much better. He'd had a great time with us, but he thought it would be better for him to stay living at his group home. I was disappointed but also a bit relieved. We both felt good knowing that the option was available, should the need arise. I wrote a story about our conundrum for the *Milwaukee Journal Sentinel,* and it caught the eye of one of Jake's old St. Francis Xavier School classmates. Jim Eberle, better known as "Ebbs," invited Jake to lunch.

Ebbs told Jake that he'd felt badly over the years about the way the boys on the playground had treated him long ago. He said he was sorry to see that Jake was having a hard time now that Holmer was dead. *Is there anything I can do for you?* Ebbs asked.

Jake thought for a bit. *Well, I do need a job,* he said.

So, Ebbs, who owns an electrical contracting company, hired him as inventory manager.

Jake loves the job. Even now, years later, Ebbs and I check in with each other to compare notes about how Jake is doing. Ebbs is always good about giving Jake time off when he needs it. He includes Jake in the company's Christmas bonus plan. During the height of the pandemic, when Jake was confined to his room for nearly a year, Ebbs petitioned the group home's management to grant Jake permission to come to work. He took pictures of all of his employees holding signs that read COME BACK, JAKE. WE MISS YOU!

You're an angel among us, I texted Ebbs after his appeal proved successful.

Ebbs pooh-poohed any heroics on his part. I need his help!!!

ONCE AGAIN, AS MY family life seemed to be back cruising on autopilot, the pressure at work was cranking into high gear. I'd been assigned to write a story that was getting more attention as the number of mass shootings increased: why it is so difficult to determine whether a person with severe mental illness is an imminent danger and how can you get them help before something tragic happens. The assignment made me nervous.

Despite the way they are often portrayed in popular culture, people with severe mental illness are rarely dangerous. In fact, they are more likely to be a victim of a violent crime than to cause one. But, as I had seen in my reporting over the years and in my own family, some people who are too sick to realize that they are ill can be a danger to themselves or others and need someplace safe to stay until they are better. As uncomfortable as it is to acknowledge that, it's equally irresponsible to ignore.

I understood the problem well and knew the heartbreaking consequences when we miss the signals of someone in imminent danger. The paramedics who pumped Nancy's stomach that afternoon in 1978 must not have thought she was in peril, or they would have taken her to the hospital. Yet just a few hours later, she threw herself in front of a train. Holmer clearly didn't think Danny was about to choke himself to death or he wouldn't have left him home alone and gone golfing that morning in 1997. No one wants to be held behind a locked door or forced to take medication that makes you groggy. But when should a person's right to autonomy yield to their safety or the safety of others?

These are not easy questions to answer, if there are any answers at all. I knew this story would be fraught with controversy, but there was no avoiding it. My job was to write about the mental health system. This is the "third rail" of mental health debates, so highly charged that you risk getting zapped by just touching it. It made me angry to hear gun rights advocates overstate the problem as they pushed for easier commitment laws over stricter gun measures. I was equally annoyed by mental health advocates who criticize any stories about dangerousness as reinforcing stereotypes. But it was my duty as a journalist to explore the issue. *Cancer loves stress,* my friend, a nurse, told me more than once. *You don't want your cancer coming back.*

I spent the next year traveling across the country interviewing people whose lives were shattered by someone who had slipped through the cracks and failed to get the care they needed: the father of Gaby Giffords' congressional aide, gunned down alongside her at a Tuscon, Arizona, shopping mall; the husband of a Virginia Tech professor who was killed with thirty-one others by a man who had ignored a court order for psychiatric care; a woman who had been desperately searching for help for her son when he stabbed her father to death during a psychotic break.

These were each deeply disturbing stories, and part of me wanted to look away. I knew it was taking an emotional toll on me, but a bigger part of me wanted to keep going, harder. We'd built up so much momentum that it would be a shame to ease off.

Now George Stanley, the managing editor, wanted me to do a deep dive into the county's mental health policies, go back—line by line—over thirty years of county budgets and policy decisions to find out why hospital administrators were making the same mistakes over and over.

My stories had already managed to anger a good number of people over the years—county administrators, nurses, even some mental health advocates who thought I focused too heavily on mismanagement and ineptitude and the sufferings of the very sickest. *Recovery is possible,* the advocates said. They wanted me to write more success stories, to give people hope. I understood their point. But I believed then that my time and energy were better spent exposing the injustices to people with serious mental illness.

Besides, George was right. The Milwaukee system was especially ripe for scrutiny, given its abysmal track record of chronically inefficient and ineffective treatment. Paid consultants had been recommending reforms for decades that went unheeded. The county was pouring most of its resources into emergency psychiatric care with little regard for preventive care or long-term treatment, the equivalent of putting a Band-Aid on a broken leg when the real problem is bone cancer.

Milwaukee County's mental health system, like systems all over the country, was no system at all but a cluster of siloed bureaucracies whose employees did not communicate well with one another. Complicating matters, Wisconsin's law requires a police officer—not a doctor—to initiate emergency mental health care even if the patient is willing to be treated. Police are not mental health care providers, nor do they want to be. Some underestimate the danger; others are too quick to reach for the handcuffs and taser guns.

Without adequate treatment options in the community, patients cycle in and out of the emergency room at alarming rates. Data I got from open records requests showed that one of every three people who were brought to the psychiatric hospital for emergency care were released and returned within ninety days. Police detained one woman a staggering 196 times in six years, an average of once every eleven days. If the definition of *insanity* is "doing the same thing over and over again and expecting different results," then Milwaukee County's mental health system was clearly out of whack.

Now, federal authorities had cited the county's psychiatric hospital five times in six years for putting patients in danger after a rash of sexual assaults and three deaths there. Milwaukee's system was failing its patients again and again, a chronic crisis.

These stories would be wonky, dense with data, statistics, and the history of flawed public policy decisions. If I was going to get anyone to care about my stories, or even just read them, I'd need to find compelling human examples, show how vulnerable human beings were harmed. That meant I'd be back staring at grieving mothers, leafing through their children's baby books as they recalled how alone and frightened they felt as their children grew sicker but no one could or would help. Many were angry and not afraid to show it. "He would have been better off dying in his crib on the day he was born," one mother told me. "It would have spared us all thirty-five years of agony."

Danny's words kept rattling around in my brain: *Only love and understanding.* Find someone who loves a person with chronic serious mental illness, and let them help you show what it's like so that readers will understand. I would need action, a little mystery, and a dash of hope to keep readers engaged. A few days later, my phone rang. Debbie Sweeney was calling. She was the answer to my prayers.

. . .

LIKE SO MANY FRUSTRATED family members, Debbie called me often over the years to complain about Milwaukee's psychiatric hospital. Her son, Rob, had been in treatment off and on for the past six years. Rob had dropped out of college in his freshman year after he started hearing voices. Police hauled him to Milwaukee County's psychiatric emergency room at least twelve times. Each time, he stayed for a few hours or a few days, depending on what he wanted or what his insurance coverage would allow, then he was back on the streets.

Rob couldn't find a landlord in Milwaukee who would rent to him anymore. He made too much noise and too much mess. He'd been kicked out of homeless shelters for breaking curfew, trashing the furniture, and ignoring the ban on smoking indoors. He was living out of motel rooms— when he could afford it and where they would allow him—with money from his federal disability account. Or he was sleeping under bushes or begging his mother to let him sleep on her couch.

Rob was doing things that made his mother sick with worry. Occasionally, he imagined people were trying to kill him. Rob once ran into a stranger's house at two o'clock in the morning, convinced he was being chased. "Thank God that family didn't pull a gun on him," Debbie said.

In the past few years, Rob had taken to keeping a knife in his pocket to keep the "evil people" away. When Debbie found a butcher knife under his bed, she told Rob that he couldn't stay at home anymore. Still, he sneaked into her house from time to time and stood by her bed late at night. Debbie started locking her bedroom door.

"That's what this disease does to you," she said. "It tears a mother away from her son."

Now, in desperation, she was taking him out to California's Silicon Valley to see if he could find a place that would take care of him and, maybe, where he could get a job someday. Her father had lived there for a time in the 1980s, so they knew how beautiful it was. "Rob's really good with computers," Debbie said.

What a compelling story for my series: a mother so frantic to get help for her son that she was turning her back entirely on our broken Milwau-kee public mental health system and traveling two thousand miles for help. *Could I come along?*

I would chronicle her odyssey, taking readers along on this ill-conceived and desperate quest. They would have a front-row seat to the drama and heartbreak of living with someone with serious mental illness.

Sure! Debbie said. Two weeks later, the three of us were off to California. It was a disaster.

WE DROVE AROUND FOR days trying to find a place that would admit Rob. He was a lot sicker than even I imagined. Like Danny, Rob was brooding and erratic and verbally abusive to his mother. I stayed in a hotel several miles away from theirs, both for my own emotional safety and to establish reasonable boundaries. Debbie couldn't help but ask for my advice from time to time. I'd made it clear that I was along with them as a journalist, not a confidante, an advocate, or a cheerleader, though it was hard to deny Debbie some moral support. She was so well-intentioned and over-whelmed, and she reminded me in some ways of my mother. They both seemed to put up with their sons' bad behavior either out of a sense of guilt or because they lacked the energy to fight back.

On the third day we were in California, Rob refused to get out of bed, calling his mother a "fucking idiot." Debbie and I took a drive to Half Moon Bay and walked along the beach, marveling at the mother sea otters playing with their pups.

"Sometimes, I feel like just running away," Debbie said. "I'd like to get in the car and drive as far as it'll take me and never come back."

Debbie wasn't the only one who was exhausted.

I just want to come home, I'd tell Larry when I'd call home at night. It was so painful to see a mother getting chewed up by her son's very serious mental illness. But I also knew this is the cost of immersive journalism, bearing witness to the tough stuff to give readers a penetrating look into issues that needed to be exposed and understood.

Against formidable odds, Debbie found a group home for Rob outside

San Jose on the last day of our twelve-day journey. "Get out of here, Mom," Rob snarled at Debbie as she kissed him goodbye. The walls of our adjoining hotel rooms that night were thin enough that I could hear Debbie crying. She and I left the next day to go back to Milwaukee, both nervous about how this would play out.

Rob lasted three nights before he was kicked out of the home for breaking curfew. Back in Milwaukee, Debbie was so discouraged that she didn't have the energy to meet him at the train station, where he was scheduled to arrive the following afternoon. So, I went to meet Rob, waiting and waiting. Unbeknownst to us, Rob had been kicked off the train in Sacramento for harassing his fellow passengers. Police found him roaming the streets several hours later and took him to the nearest psychiatric hospital.

Two days later, Debbie and I flew back to California to fetch him. It was as grim an assignment as I'd ever been on. Rob was significantly sicker-looking and -acting than when we first took off for California. Debbie was all that and several thousands of dollars poorer.

The next month, Debbie went on disability from her job. Her arms and legs ached. She could barely get out of bed.

"I was becoming very forgetful and crying all the time," she said.

She spent most of her days lying on the couch.

"I thought this would give me some peace, to know that I tried," she said. "But it's not enough. I actually think I made Rob's life worse." A few weeks after that, Debbie checked herself into the psychiatric unit of a nearby hospital, saying she felt like killing herself.

Not surprisingly, I was having a tough time writing this story. I'd written it like a diary, but some of the editors thought it was too dark, that it rambled, the way living with severe mental illness can feel. They were right. But I had hit a wall, and it was hard to think clearly about how to write this. Greg Borowski, the hardworking, soft-spoken investigations editor, told me it should not be too much work to revise the copy. Still, I snapped.

I can't work on this anymore, I told myself. *I don't have one more ounce of energy in my body. I just want this to be over. Now.* I threw my notebook across the newsroom and stormed out of the building. I wasn't angry at

Greg; I was furious at the situation, feeling out of control. For the next hour or so, I felt like I was floating outside of my own body. I marched to my car and turned the engine on with no idea where I was going.

AN HOUR LATER, I was lying on the beach in the sand with my feet in the water, staring at the sky. I'd driven north of downtown Milwaukee to a park called the Lion's Den. Still in a kind of trance, I scrambled through the forest and down the steps to the shores of Lake Michigan, where I dropped to my knees.

As I lay there, I considered how my campaign to humiliate public officials into improving mental health care had crumbled. *Your stories aren't saving people. In fact, they might be making them sicker,* I told myself. *Poor Debbie is in the hospital. Rob is even sicker than when you left for California a month ago.* What role had I played in that? Had I been so enamored with the adventurous story line that I'd lost sight of the consequences to these two? How had it helped them to have the intimate details of their traumatic trip splayed across the front page of the daily newspaper?

Journalists love tidy story lines. We embrace the role of crusader, hoping that the light we shine on a problem will be powerful enough to disinfect it. *Comfort the afflicted. Afflict the comfortable!* my editors and I are fond of saying. This was the ethos that fueled me throughout my life. When Patty and I were young and would get into a fight, I'd pin her down on the ground and yell into her ear: *Admit defeat!* That's what I was hoping my stories would do. Overpower policy makers with the truth. Shock readers into action the way activists like Dorothea Dix and muckrakers like Nellie Bly, Ida Tarbell, and Albert Deutsch had done when they exposed the horrific conditions of insane asylums.

Sometimes, it worked. My stories on the horrible housing conditions had led to hundreds of new units being built. But, as I was now learning, making life better for people with serious mental illness is not as simple as shaming others into providing housing, more doctors, better medications. If the change is going to be real and sustained, you can't just badger people into being better, more loving and accepting. You have to find a way to get them to see those who suffer as their brothers and sisters in need of our embrace, not strangers to be shunned. It's what Danny was trying to tell me in the letter he sent me the week before he died.

Only love and understanding can conquer this disease.

My grand scheme had been a failure. I was beat up and drained of energy, lying on the shore like a washed-up alewife. I wasn't going to get my readers to love and understand people with mental illness by beating them over the head with these disturbing stories. I'd have to go deeper, find a new way to tell the story.

You can't keep doing this, I told myself. *You're going to crack up, and you might not be able to pull yourself together again this time.*

HOLMER'S WIFE DIED IN September 2014. One of her daughters called Jake three days later to let him know. I wondered if they were keeping the news from us so that we wouldn't come to the wake and funeral, but Mary Kay thought that sounded a little cynical. As it turned out, his wife indeed had pulled something of a switcheroo. She wasn't going to be cremated as she and Holmer had planned after all. Instead, she would be buried next to her first husband with her portion of Holmer's ashes tucked inside her casket.

Other betrayals would soon follow. A few months after our stepmother's funeral, Mary Kay was driving around Wilmette when she saw a sign for an estate sale at a familiar address: Holmer's old condominium. Her children were selling our family belongings without any notice to us. If that wasn't bad enough, Mary Kay realized, as she pulled into the parking lot, the sale had started the day before. The professional organizer would not let her inside. *But my mother's furniture is in there,* Mary Kay said, standing at the door. *Those belonged to our grandparents and great-grandparents.* The man would not be swayed. *Sorry,* he said. *No family permitted.*

We didn't have a legal leg to stand on. Holmer, the old lawyer, had updated his will a few years before he died, bequeathing any earthly possessions he hadn't already liquidated to his wife. That included my mother's family treasures—some old mahogany furniture, the few silver-plated pieces they hadn't already sold, and some bone china.

We'd been afraid that something like this might happen. A month or so after Holmer died, our aunt Dodie, the widow of my mother's brother, Tom, took his wife to an expensive restaurant, hoping that, if she buttered her up enough, the wife would see it in her heart to give us some of the Gutenkunst family belongings. *They're really only interested in some things of their mother's,* my aunt said. The wife told Aunt Dodie that she was too distraught about Holmer's death to concentrate on details like that. She'd need time to think about it. *If I decide to give them anything, I'll let Mary Kay know.* But she never did.

Now Mary Kay was getting the boot as she tried to retrieve anything that we considered a family heirloom. So I dispatched my old St. Francis pal Terry to buy up all she could of whatever was left of our childhood chattel. Patty did the same with a few of her friends. They sent texts of themselves in funny hats sipping imaginary tea from the newly ransomed china.

For a couple hundred bucks, we came away with my great-grandparents' nightstand, some mismatched water goblets, and a few place settings of Wedgwood dishes. These sentimental treasures may not have been worth much on the open market, but they represented pieces of our past, and it was painful to see them sold to strangers without our consent. As with Holmer's ashes and the family pictures that had been schlepped to the rummage sale years earlier, the crude disposal of my mother's family belongings felt like another kick in the gut, like the things we valued were little more than garbage.

This is from your grandmother, I told my daughter, Molly, misty-eyed, at her wedding shower a few months later as I handed her a box with one of my mother's Wedgwood teacups and saucers. Molly was just four years old when my mother died, but I knew she would treasure this tangible link to her grandmother. All she remembered of my mother came from snapshots and a grainy home movie of her putting nail polish on Molly's little fingers. Molly smiled as she examined the delicate white and blue ivy pattern. When she turned the cup over, I saw her face fall. *Oops,* I said. *Give me that thing.* I grabbed the cup quickly and peeled off the neon tag that advertised a sale price of two dollars.

After losing Nancy and Danny, my mother, and Holmer, it felt a little petty to be stewing over salad plates and some silver tongs. *Get off the pity pot!* I could practically hear Holmer shouting from his multiple graves. He would be right. The real treasures, of course, could not be sold at a discount.

The six of us Kissingers still had each other.

WITH MY EDITORS' DEFT oversight, I finished my yearlong examination of the county's troubled mental health system. The series had been an un-qualified success, prompting reforms of state law. It was declared a winner by the judges of the George Polk Award as a "revelatory, analytical and conclusive study of a system that barely functions."

But now I was the one barely functioning.

My nerves felt shot. I'd run out of energy. I was starting to get flash-backs:

My mother's wrist, bandaged where she tried to open her veins with a pair of scissors.

Nancy's casket swinging on the crane.

The handwritten note that Danny stuffed into his pocket just before wrapping the electrical cord around his neck, urging him to "collect trea-sures for Heaven."

I wanted a break from waking up each morning and thinking about these things and about how to quantify the harm to people whose brains betrayed them. But I didn't have the courage to say so. Was it my ego? Guilt? A savior complex? Or was I, just like any reporter on a hot beat, a dog with a bone?

Out of the blue came an opportunity for a fresh start. I'd been offered positions as a visiting professor, first at my alma mater in Indiana, then at Columbia University's Graduate School of Journalism in New York City, teaching investigative reporting. Susanne, my old newsroom reporting partner, was supervising a team of Columbia science journalism fellows and recommended me to the dean. I jumped at the chance.

Here was a new way for me to attack the same old beast—training bright young reporters with a lot more energy and data skills than I had to expose the cracks in the so-called mental health system. Many of them had struggled with their own mental health or had close relatives who did. They shared my enthusiasm for shining a light on this scandal. Some were eager to share the details of their battles with depression, eating disorders, and anxiety. As grateful and impressed as I was with their candor, I didn't want my class to be regarded as a kind of group therapy session.

My job was to train them to conduct skillful investigations of why people aren't getting the care they need, to identify specifically who is responsible, and, if possible, to suggest solutions.

Investigative reporting is tough enough, I told them. But writing about people with mental illness is especially challenging. "No one cares about crazy people," that awful Wisconsin political operative had said in reaction to our stories about the dangerous conditions inside the Milwaukee County Mental Health Complex. Unfortunately, she's not the only one who believes that. If we were writing about celebrities or abused animals, you'd have no trouble getting internet traffic, I told my students. But the fact of the matter is that many people with a lifetime of serious mental illness, rich in their humanity as they may be, look pretty banged up. They don't make appealing clickbait.

Besides, readers can be fickle, I warned them. Many have the attention span of a hummingbird. There are lots of other things they're more interested in than the plight of someone with depression or schizophrenia.

Find a way to make people care. Get to know the subjects of your stories, beyond the labels of their particular illness. Spend time with them. Sit down, shut up, and let them talk. Find out what they like to eat, what frightens them, what makes them laugh, what they wanted to do with their lives before their illness grabbed them by the throat. Go where the people are.

Huddle with families in community centers, church basements, mosques, and synagogues and listen to them weep as they recall how mental illness transformed a person they loved into someone they could no longer recognize. Ride along with the police, as I did in Memphis and Houston and Milwaukee, to see how they treat someone in the middle of a psychotic break. Take readers into their world like a correspondent embedded in a war zone.

Get them to see the world the way that your subjects do, feel what they are feeling. Then describe that with such precision that your readers feel it, too.

I was lucky enough to have editors who supported my travels. My reporting took me all over, from New York to San Jose, Pittsburgh, Chicago, Columbus, San Antonio, Austin, Sacramento, San Francisco, even tiny Geel, Belgium, where, for more than seven hundred years, the people of the town have housed and cared for people with severe mental illness.

Here's the trickiest part of writing about people with mental illness:

Tempting as it is to want to help the people that we write about, we are not their advocates. Leave that to organizations like the National Alliance on Mental Illness and Mental Health America. Our responsibility is to tell the story, to educate readers. We shine the light; they try to solve the problem.

Still, you often can't help but care about the people you cover, especially the more intimately you get to know them, I said. Stories can take months, sometimes years. You get to know your subjects very well. I thought about John Spoerl, Georgia Rawlings, Jim Hankin, Debbie Sweeney, and so many of the hundreds of others I'd written about in the past three decades. I'd come to see them in much deeper, more layered and complex ways than the people I wrote about on my other beats. The more I got to know them, the greater I cared about each of them.

"To be a great journalist, you have to be willing to be wounded by the stories you tell," I said, quoting a talk that Pope Francis gave honoring two longtime Vatican reporters. Then, I added a twist of my own: You need to find a way to let those broken hearts mend. Don't let yourself get sucked in and chewed up. *It's quite a high-wire act.*

. . .

AS I TAUGHT THEM, I found that I was educating myself, too, psyching my-self up to take on the one story that I'd been too afraid to tell, the one that haunted me for years. The one that hurt too much to think about, the one I knew I'd need to report if I was ever going to find peace about my past.

My siblings and I told ourselves repeatedly over the years that there was nothing more we could have done to save Nancy and Danny. If they wanted to die badly enough, they would find a way. That's what Holmer kept telling us, and that made us feel better, but was it really true?

Suicide prevention experts I'd interviewed over the years told me re-peatedly that we can do a lot more to stop people from killing themselves. Knowing the warning signs for suicide and how to talk to those who are considering it will save lives. So, why weren't we able to stop our siblings, especially Danny?

Because we had been discouraged from talking about it, I never took the time to deeply consider if there was more we could have done. For years, the mystery ate away at me.

Had the mishandling of one family tragedy laid the groundwork for others?

So many times over the years, I could not help but wonder what life would have been like if we had grown up in a more transparent era, one that would not have encouraged us to hide our mother's mysterious ab-sences or our father's violent outbursts. What if we hadn't been driven to secrecy by our embarrassment about Nancy's death? How would things have been different if we'd been encouraged to consider her illness—all our family's illnesses—in more straightforward, nonjudgmental ways? If Nancy and Danny had died of leukemia or a heart defect, we'd be scram-bling to learn all we could about those diseases, to protect ourselves from the same fate. We wouldn't be turning away from one another in shame. I needed to know, or at least try to know, where and how things went wrong so that the next time someone thought about jumping in front of a train or wrapping an electric cord around their neck, we could be there to help.

What if we had not been so ashamed?

No doubt we would have been more vigilant when Mary Kay went into one of her occasional funks, when Jake started having trouble sleeping, when I began lashing out in anger at the slightest annoyance. We could have helped when Patty started looking paler and thinner. When Billy's panic attacks began. When Danny started obsessing over his blood sugar levels. When Molly moved to the mountains with a stash of weed but without a phone number for us to reach her. If we'd been taught about the warning signs of mental illness or even just the language to talk about it, we would have been better equipped to care for one another, or at the very least, to offer comfort.

Reporters reverse engineer disasters all the time. 9/11. George Floyd's murder. The January 6 insurrection. We break down the sequence of events leading up to them and look for cracks in the system, inflection points where one decision could have averted the tragedies. We try to identify the flaws in the system, hoping that they will be corrected so something so terrible won't happen again. This is what I wanted to do with my family's story, go back over the events of the days that Nancy and Danny died—and the months and years leading up to them—to see if there was anything more we could have done to change the outcome.

I hoped that the lessons of what we went through could help others. At the very least, our story could be a kind of candle in the window for those who have lost a family member to suicide. If we shared our story, they could see that they are not alone.

For more than two decades, I'd looked to strangers to tell the story of how and why people with mental illness are not getting the care they need. Now it was time to turn the notebook on my family and me. I wanted to show as unflinchingly as possible what the long-term consequences are when you are shamed into silence. Not to browbeat but to bear witness.

This was either the greatest or stupidest story idea of my life.

PART III

❖

Letting Go

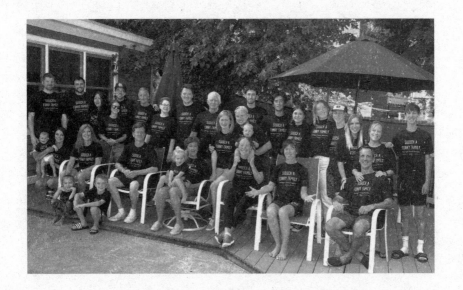

17

Like Sparks Through Stubble

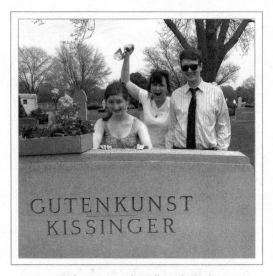

Mother's Day with Molly and Charley,
Holy Cross Cemetery, Milwaukee, Wisconsin, 2014.

The immortal words of Marion G. Harmon kept ringing in my ears as I set out to investigate our family's story: "Everything happens for a reason. Sometimes, the reason is that you're stupid and make bad decisions."

For this to work, I'd need buy-in from each of my brothers and sisters. I was not interested in writing a sanitized version of our family history or a memoir by committee, but I wasn't willing to sacrifice my relationships with any of them either. We'd already lost too much.

No one knew what my reporting might yield. That made me anxious. I'd be looking through my mother's diaries and Holmer's AA books and examining any medical files of theirs that I could locate. I also hoped to find Nancy's and Danny's medical records and the police and coroner's reports from their suicides. Of course, I could not tell the full story of our family without including the details from Danny's hate mail trial forty years earlier. Resurrecting that humiliation would be difficult for everyone, particularly those of us with spouses, in-laws, children, and grandchildren who are Jewish. So, if any one of my siblings said they were opposed to me writing about this, the deal was off.

As I had hoped, no one hesitated. Not even a little bit. They were just as invested as I was in the hope that telling our family's story could help others. As I collected the evidence, I put what I found in a common internet file so that they could access the information if they chose to do so.

I'd need their help to remember some of the details from so many years ago. They each responded to my phone calls, emails, and texts, sometimes at crazy hours, often about something painful to recall. It felt sometimes like we were playing a warped game of Trivial Pursuit, Kissinger Family–Style. *Did Mom cut her wrist that Christmas with scissors or her knitting needles? What year and where was Holmer arrested for drunk driving?*

Then there were the real gut punchers: Had we done enough to help each other? Do you ever worry that we might be doomed by our genetics? What trauma or mental illnesses might we have passed along to the next generation?

To execute this plan soundly, I would need lots of scaffolding. In other words, therapy. My track record in this department was terrible. Aside from interviewing mental health experts for my newspaper articles, I'd been in a therapist's office exactly once, nearly twenty years earlier, and it didn't end well. I chickened out. My brothers and sisters had been smart enough to get professional help decades earlier, but I was still clinging to Drink, Pray, Swim, my do-it-yourself mental health regimen, a poor woman's version of Eat, Pray, Love.

Now that I was plowing through this minefield of our family's past, I didn't trust myself to do this on my own anymore. Too risky. I knew I would need a therapist trained in trauma to help me get to those deeper truths as I managed my relationships with my family.

The first therapist I chose was one I found surfing the web who matched my less than exacting requirements—she took my insurance and looked friendly. Our relationship was doomed from the start.

That was my fault. I cast these meetings like a story assignment. I was the reporter, and she was my source. Once again, I could hide behind my reporter's notebook so I didn't have to deal with my own feelings. I was in the driver's seat and had it all under control, or so I told myself. So, I never really opened up. And she didn't probe. After meeting for a few months, it was clear that this was not helping me frame the tough questions I needed to ask. What more could we have done to save Nancy and Danny?

Good news: my therapist has shingles! I texted a former student, now friend, who had encouraged me to try therapy. While I did not wish this very nice therapist any harm, her illness was a good excuse to wiggle away and find someone who would be a better fit for me.

I found Kate on a recommendation from a friend. Kate had read my newspaper articles over the years and believed, as I did, that there was value in examining all that I could about what had happened to me and my family. We both hoped that I would heal and grow and that others could learn from us. I worried that some of this was ancient history, too much scar tissue, too difficult to summon. But the longer I worked with Kate, the more I learned that it's never too late to reckon with your past. But, brace yourself: it is going to be painful.

She would help me make sense of what happened and put it into perspective. We worked to understand what has changed and what has not. This time, I promised myself that I would surrender to the process and trust her as my ally and guide.

Kate was on to me from day one. She could see right away that I was quick to redirect the conversation when the pain got too intense by either offering a sassy retort or an apology. We'd have to scrape off fifty years of denials and excuses and my people-pleasing/bullshitting ways.

So many of my reflexes were working against me to get to the bottom of this story. Grandma and the nuns had admonished me to quit my bellyaching—*Offer it up to the poor souls in purgatory!* As a reporter, I'd been trained to keep myself out of my stories. *Just the facts, ma'am.* As a Kissinger, I resorted to dark humor to ease the sting. Tragedy + more tragedy = comedy. *No laughing in the fucking suicide line!*

But now I'd have to sit with these most painful memories and all that I was learning from the evidence I was gathering. I'd need to let it marinate and see what lessons I could derive. How has all this trauma affected me and my siblings?

Listen to what you are saying, Kate often says. *Write that down!*

I sent Kate the first two chapters of my book, and for the next few years, we would meet every other week or so to be sure that I was able to absorb what I was discovering. Our goal was for me to not become overwhelmed by any of my usual reactions: sadness, anger, fear, regret, and—God help me—more shame. I'd been taking emotional shortcuts for more than a half century—steam-cleaning, beer drinking, and smart-assing my way through one trauma after another. But I was learning that you can't fast-forward through grief or read a CliffsNotes version of your life and expect to make peace with it. As I revisited old memories, I allowed my new feelings to surface and hang around long enough to acknowledge and try to reconcile. Almost immediately, I could see that so much of my family narrative as I had understood it was either woefully incomplete or just flat-out wrong.

The most surprising and, for me, the most telling detail I learned was that, contrary to my long-held belief, my mother was *not* at home on that Friday afternoon in June 1978 when Nancy slipped out the back door and headed toward the train tracks. The story I'd either been told—or just assumed—was that she was in the basement doing laundry and didn't hear the door slam shut when Nancy left. Because we never did family therapy or talked as a group about that day, we each carried our own version of the events. It was only decades later, after I collected the various accounts from each of my brothers and sisters, that the fuller, more disturbing story emerged.

I always feared that I had contributed to Nancy's death. When I called home from my receptionist job at the downtown marketing agency late that morning to tell my mother that I would not be coming home that night, I had no idea that Nancy had just swallowed a bottle's worth of sleeping pills. She sounded groggy and snarky, but she often sounded that way, especially to me. For years, I felt guilty about how I'd talked to my sister that day, calling her out for being rude. I worried that I'd only made Nancy feel worse about herself and that I contributed to her decision to do what she was about to do. Turns out, I was far from the only one racked with guilt about Nancy's final hours.

People are at the highest risk of suicide just after they have made an attempt. Nancy should have been under intense surveillance that day. Patty knew that, which was why she'd offered to get out of her waitressing shift and stay at home.

Just go, our mother told Patty. *I'll watch her.*

But she didn't. My mother left, putting thirteen-year-old Molly in charge.

Molly had just graduated from eighth grade. She had been on her way home earlier that day when she saw the ambulance in our driveway and decided to turn her bike around and steer her way clear of that mess. Even at that young age, Molly knew from experience that there wasn't anything she could do in these situations but stand there and stare, and she'd seen enough.

Molly returned home at around 3:30 that afternoon, assuming that any commotion caused by Nancy's latest suicide attempt must have died down by then. She planned to hang out for a while and watch TV until it was time to get ready for her 5 p.m. graduation party a few blocks down, one that our parents were co-hosting. As Molly walked in the house, my mother asked her to keep an eye on Nancy so she could go out for a bit. No one can say for sure where our mother went that day. But it was a Friday afternoon, and she always—*always*—went to the hairdresser on Friday afternoons.

Nancy, despite having tried to kill herself less than three hours earlier, was now being supervised by a child not old enough to babysit by Illinois law.

Molly checked in on Nancy a few times that afternoon and found her asleep each time. She didn't linger, repulsed by the smell of Nancy's vomit.

My mother returned home at about 4:45 p.m. and went upstairs to check on Nancy. Her bed was empty. Molly and my mother looked all over the house for her, unaware that, as they searched from room to room, Nancy was stumbling toward the train tracks three blocks to the west.

Just go to your party, my mother told Molly. *I will see you there later.*

As Molly walked out the door, she heard my mother calling the police to report that Nancy was missing. A few minutes later, Molly heard the sirens blare.

"Lots and lots of sirens," Molly recalled years later. She cringed. "I figured they were for Nancy."

Still, she kept walking.

I was flabbergasted when Molly explained how my mother had foisted the responsibility for watching Nancy on her. What kind of mother puts a thirteen-year-old child in that position, knowing, as she did, how intent Nancy had been on killing herself just a few hours earlier? The same kind of mother who leaves her kids in the toy department so she can go Christmas shopping. The same kind of mother who lets one toddler after another wander out of the house, to the pier, the state highway, the witchy old lady's house down the block. The same kind of mother who lets her daughter know that her grandmother is dead by leaving a two-word message with the college dorm receptionist. WHILE MY MOTHER WAS OUT . . . Nancy jumped in front of a train.

My blood started to boil. I was so angry that I felt like I might explode. Poor Patty! Poor Molly! Poor Nancy! My mother had been dead for more than twenty-five years by the time I learned this. It was too late to ask her for an explanation. How do you argue with a ghost? I would have to try to understand her motivations as best I could without ever really knowing the truth. The deeper I delved into my mother's life, the clearer I understood.

She may not have talked about them, but my mother had demons of her own. The more I considered her life story, the more I could see that she was overwhelmed. We'd always joked about how she was "spacy like a fox," how deftly she could tune out some of our wildest antics and still sort the laundry with military precision. (Let the record show that not once did I get the wrong pair of underwear or socks in my laundry pile.) I'd never paused to understand what it must have been like for my mother to raise all those kids more or less on her own, with her own paralyzing bouts of depression and anxiety and a husband who often was absent, drunk, or out of control.

No doubt my mother was upset that day, having just watched Nancy try to kill herself again. How many times had Nancy attempted suicide at that point? Ten? Eleven? We'd lost count. My mother had no way to know whether Nancy really meant to kill herself by swallowing those pills. Was she taking a risk by leaving the house later that day? Absolutely. But I see now why she felt that she couldn't keep putting her obligations on hold to monitor Nancy 24-7. She needed to take care of herself, run her errands, even get her hair done, if that's where she was that afternoon. Such a seemingly reckless decision should not be considered in a vacuum.

The empty vodka bottles that my mother stashed in the back of her closet in the years after Nancy died are testimony to how guilty she must have felt about leaving that day. I couldn't judge her any harsher than she'd already judged herself. If I was going to move on, I'd need to find a way to forgive my mother, just as she had forgiven me for my many faults and misdeeds over the years. She was so much more than this one tragic decision. "I miss you like crazy," she'd written to me in the early days of my first newspaper job. "We all do."

Nor did I know that Patty had become so depressed in the years that followed that she checked herself into a psychiatric hospital for a few days during her senior year of college. I had just started my new job in Cincinnati at that time and was focused on making a good impression on my editors. Patty and I talked, but not about Nancy. I knew she felt guilty about going to work that day, but I didn't help her see that it was not her fault that Nancy died. The idea of my little Tiger Pit pal suffering like that brought me to tears, even after so many decades.

Remembering this now, Patty is fuzzy on the details. She can't recall the name of the hospital where she was treated or which nursing instructor helped check her into the psych ward. She wished she could, so that she could thank her.

"She probably saved my life," Patty said.

Milwaukee's troubled mental health system had been my beat for more than twenty years, but I never knew that my beloved sister Patty had been one of the patients. Or that the staff had helped her to get better. I hunted down an old faculty directory from that era, but Patty still could not conjure the name.

"I wish I could, but that's how out of it I was," Patty said.

It scared me to hear Patty say that she lost control of herself.

"I don't know if I would have killed myself, but I might have. I wasn't thinking straight," Patty said.

Though so many years had passed, just the thought of Patty considering suicide made me feel like I was choking. I'm still not sure which is more disturbing—that Patty was so vulnerable then or that I had no idea that she was. The power of shame can get between even the closest of sisters.

Patty says she still feels guilty about going to work that day.

"I probably always will," she said.

Mercifully, Molly had managed to come to terms about her role that day years ago. "I was a kid!" she said. But it wasn't easy for her. Years of therapy, mindfulness, and meditation helped Molly to understand that Nancy's suicide was not her fault. I wish that she and Patty had talked to each other about this years earlier so that Patty could have been spared so much remorse, too.

Secrets can strangle relationships. For fifty years, Mary Kay had been tortured by her decision to have an abortion. I wish I could have comforted her, but we never talked about it.

She told me the details in 2021. Until then, I never knew about the effort that it took for Mary Kay to get to New York City and back without any of us learning about it. As she described her ordeal to me, I tried to imagine what it must have been like for her, barely nineteen years old, walking into our dark, empty house that night in 1971, bleeding and scared. Here was yet another example of how our secrets and unresolved trauma might have proved to be deadly.

"Over the years, I have felt such shame in having to keep yet another secret from people I loved because of the taboos that surround abortion," Mary Kay wrote to me in an email. "With the mental illness and substance abuse in our family, this was just another secret to be kept."

In hindsight, Mary Kay's retreat from our family made perfect sense. She was in pain, and being around all of us made her feel dirty, sinful, and ashamed and, ultimately, angry. "I often felt I would explode from all the things I had experienced and couldn't share and mourn with anyone else," she said.

My heart broke for her thinking how lonely she was holding all of that inside. While I was relieved that Mary Kay finally found a way to talk about her feelings, I worried about whether she wanted to reveal them here and risk the wrath of those who only see the world in black and white.

But her trauma is an important part of our family story. I admire her bravery in coming forward so others can understand what it is like for a young woman with severe depression to be faced with an unplanned pregnancy. She'd seriously considered suicide. Ultimately, she chose what she considered to be her only good option.

"These are memories that I have stuffed down for fifty years," Mary Kay said.

Reliving them was not easy.

"I actually felt the same anxiety, fear, shame, regret, anger, and a dark black sadness from all those years ago," Mary Kay said. "I would sometimes have physical reactions and would have to stop and walk around or do deep breathing to calm down. I guess some of this shit never goes away."

Still, she thanked me for asking her to talk about it. Once she was able to go back and thoughtfully consider those days with the help of her therapist, Nora, Mary Kay was finally able to understand her choice more clearly and make peace with it.

"In steering me back to that time, I have been forced to look at the girl I was then and, knowing what I do about myself now, be able to reframe and understand why I did this," she said.

Learning Mary Kay's story made me realize even more how vulnerable we each had been and how important it is to wrestle with your past so you can learn to let go.

These days, Mary Kay is making up for lost time with the rest of us. She's the first to send a birthday text, organize a family barbecue, or volunteer to go with Jake to one of his doctor appointments.

OPEN RECORDS LAWS NOTWITHSTANDING, I had to really dig to get the Wilmette Police to send the reports of Nancy's and Danny's deaths. At first, they told me they were no longer available. I knew that couldn't be true. As it turned out, the public information officer just didn't know where to look for them. Ultimately, the police chief sent them to me in an email with an apology.

I was nervous about opening the files, even though so many years had gone by—twenty-two since Danny died and almost twice as long for Nancy. I took a deep breath and clicked the button. Though I'd been exposed to my share of gore and grisly details in my time covering night cops and criminal courts at *The Cincinnati Post* and *The Milwaukee Journal,* I've always been something of a wimp when it comes to dead bodies, especially ones I'm related to. But I felt I had to comb through the reports if I was going to have some closure.

My imagination had taken me to some crazy places over the years as I wondered precisely how my sister and brother died and what they were thinking in the moments leading up to their deaths. I had been haunted by a study that found that nearly half of all people who survived a suicide attempt made their decision within the previous ten minutes, and most were glad that their attempt had failed. Could one of us have stopped Nancy or Danny? I decided that I would rather know the truth than continue to consider even worse possibilities.

What I found gave me strange comfort.

Nancy was not lying on the tracks, as I had imagined for years. She was running along the middle of them to make certain that she would be hit. Likewise, Danny was not dangling from the electrical cord that he had wrapped around his neck, the way I had always pictured it. He was on his knees at the bottom of the stairs, leaning into the cord. He could have stopped himself at any time. Clearly, they both wanted to die.

In an odd way, knowing that they were both so intentional about the ways they chose to kill themselves gave me peace and exonerated the guilt I had assigned myself and others. It would have been much more disturbing if we learned that Danny or Nancy had made impetuous decisions, actions we might have been able to interrupt, ones that they would later thank us for stopping.

There was one detail in the police report on Danny's death so intimate and heartbreaking that it made me gasp. I still cry sometimes when I think of it. When the cops came down the basement stairs that afternoon, they found Holmer lying on top of Danny's body, sobbing, "Why? Why?" Holmer had desperately tried to save Danny. He told the officers that he was attempting to breathe life back into Danny the way he'd done for me when I fell off the pier in Land O' Lakes decades earlier.

For years, we had all been so angry with Holmer for playing golf that morning, despite knowing how vulnerable Danny was. *Why did you leave him alone?* we asked over and over, clenching our fists. We were hurt and confused by how quickly Holmer seemed to write off Danny's death as inevitable. Reading this detail in the police file helped me to see the real story.

He wasn't callous; he was crushed. Holmer had been shattered by Danny's death. His decision to move on now seemed braver, less cavalier. That's what he'd done all his life. The same guy who was so young that he needed his parents' permission to join the navy after his brother had been killed was now showing us that we needed to pick ourselves up and keep moving, too.

Since moving to New York in recent years to teach at Columbia University, I've retraced Holmer's steps along Fifth Avenue, imagining him strutting past Cartier and Tiffany and his beloved Brooks Brothers—Mr. Big Shot with his outsized hopes and dreams. I picture him ordering a Scotch and soda at the Bull and Bear or a stinger at the Oyster Bar at Grand Central Terminal. He'd down one and then another, and another. I think about him jogging through Central Park to burn off his hangovers, and ultimately ducking into St. Patrick's Cathedral, his dreams now shattered, desperate for direction, lighting a candle, saying a prayer, taking a seat at a noontime AA meeting.

Holmer's old AA book reads like a little window into his soul.

"Honesty! Honesty!!!" he wrote. "I can't take myself too seriously."

Alcohol had taken over his life, he wrote.

Everything became affected by it.
Bad decisions
Loneliness
Guilt
Depression.

After Holmer was diagnosed with stage IV melanoma, I tried to lighten the atmosphere in the room with a little joke. It's exactly what Holmer would have done to any one of us. *Well, at least you can drink again!* He didn't laugh.

Now, staring at those pages with the words he scratched on the side of the page, I could see why.

I am sober today! Thank God and AA

Holmer kept three pieces of paper tucked into that book, a tome more precious to him than any Bible: a telephone number of his sponsor from the night he was arrested for drunk driving in New Jersey in 1976 and two notes, both from me. One was the goofy poem I had written just before Nancy died, the one I handed to him as her wake was about to begin. The other was a cartoon that I had drawn for him years later wishing him success on his bar exam. "Go, Holmer, go! Do Your Best on Your Test!!!! Get an 'A'!!!!"

My last ten years with Holmer had been so strained. I had been disgusted with him for the selfish decisions he and his wife had made—commandeering Jake's credit card, flitting to Europe and Hawaii and Palm Springs on credit they knew was no good. *What a phony!* Worse than that: *What a thief!*

As I read my poem and the little cartoon, I remembered what a cheerleader he had been for me and for all of us. Whenever one of us stumbled—a lost job, a kid in trouble at school, a fizzled romance—Holmer would call to recite his favorite saying: *It's okay to be disappointed, but don't get discouraged.*

I thought about that winter day in 1980 when Holmer went out of his way to visit me in upstate New York, how we marched through the woods on our cross-country skis, not knowing the proper technique but giving it our best.

Keep chugging, Muggs!

The more time I took to consider the trauma we had all been through, the easier I understood that two seemingly contradictory truths can exist simultaneously. My parents could be warm and loving but also reckless and flawed. Our family life could have been happy despite the tragedies.

People are a lot more complicated and nuanced than I had given them credit for. I found an old typewritten note that Holmer's father, my Grandpa Matt, sent to my mother in 1963, around the time that she was hospitalized when I was just starting first grade. He encouraged her to call him "the first time you see any place where I can help you, Bill, or the children." Apparently, my mother had confided to him how troubled she was, probably about Holmer's drinking and his volatile employment situation. Grandpa, who once scared me by threatening to cram a milk bottle down Grandma's throat, was reaching out to ease my mother's mind and help with all of us.

I thought about how Grandpa had survived his heart attack in 1943 and lived another twenty-nine years after Uncle Jack was killed. I wondered if Grandpa felt guilty that summoning his son to be by his side may have played a role in Jack's death. And yet, he found a way to keep moving forward and help others. "Things will move from now on," Grandpa wrote to his daughter-in-law. "You watch and see."

Even Grandma looked more sympathetic once I learned her backstory. I thought about how she must have felt when she learned that her son had been killed, the one she had been so cruel to. I was haunted by the specter of her shrieking so loudly that the neighbors down the block could hear her. I see now that the shame of her unresolved guilt and the trauma from her son's death must have rattled her every day. It was hard to write her off as a batty old shrew after that.

Of all the documents I found, the letters that Danny wrote to the judge hit me the hardest. None of us knew anything about them and we likely never would have had it not been for my timely email to Danny's lawyer, Mike Byrne. Mike, my old high school beer-drinking buddy, was about to toss out Danny's case files when I wrote to tell him about this book. Mike and his friend Jim also helped me to be declared as guardian of Nancy's estate so that I could get access to her medical records.

We all knew that Danny's role in harassing the truck repair shop owner and the years he spent trying to claim his innocence had taken a toll on him. But these letters showed the depth of his torment in excruciating detail. Toxicity had turned his unresolved guilt into anger and paranoia. Danny spent his whole adult life in the shadow of his hateful act. As I retyped his letters, I saw how sick my brother had become and how dangerous his thinking was.

I tried to imagine how exhausting it would be for Danny to be hiding in shame all those years. Did he always wonder if this new customer or that cute woman sitting next to him at the bar knew about this dark chapter from his past? How differently would Danny's life have turned out if he had just admitted to doing this stupid, cruel act when he was eighteen years old, asked for forgiveness, and accepted his punishment?

Instead, he spent years trying to cover it up or make increasingly thin excuses for it. Danny's inability to reconcile with his past had stunted his emotional growth and robbed him of any chance to be happy. He'd lost everything he had—his job, a few romances, his ability to live independently, even his best childhood friends.

So when Danny sat down to write to me on that August day in 1997, he had nothing left to lose. He had searched his soul and admitted that he had made a mess of his life. Finally, the truth would set him free. He pledged to take his medication, go to therapy, and do what he could to get well.

But, by then, it was too late.

. . .

NANCY'S DOCTORS, INCLUDING THE one she almost married, are all dead now. But through the miracle of the internet, I tracked down one of the social workers from her 1976 stay at Chicago-Read Mental Health Center. The woman's signature was on the notes that described Nancy as "needy and manipulative" that I had found to be so insensitive (and also true). Ursula was ninety-one years old when I called her in the summer of 2022 as she was making a pot of spaghetti in her Chicago apartment. She said she didn't remember Nancy specifically but she would be happy to talk to me about what it was like working in the state psychiatric hospital in those days.

Most of the patients were from poor or blue-collar families. "We didn't have many from Wilmette," Ursula said. That made me wonder if she might have judged Nancy more harshly, knowing that she was from a wealthy area and had so many privileges that the other patients did not.

I asked her why she would have remarked that Nancy was needy. She denied writing that. I found another note that she also signed that said Nancy "tends to say all the right things without really any conviction or understanding. She plays the 'poor me' helpless role." I wondered how she knew what Nancy's convictions were and that she was being insincere. Aren't most people in a locked psych ward needy? Isn't that why they are there? They need care! Ursula said she didn't remember writing that either.

I wasn't out to confront her or expose her to public scrutiny. I just wanted a better understanding of how patients were treated then.

"We didn't do much therapy in those days," she said. "We just gave the patients lots of medication and let them sleep. You'd be surprised by how often that's all they needed."

Like Patty, they would go home a few days later and never return again. Ursula told me she was a social worker there from 1975 to 2011. She said she wanted to write a book of her own someday about all the "crazy people who worked at that place." Then she asked me if I knew the joke about the difference between mental patients and psychiatrists. (Answer: The doctors have the keys.) "Well, we used to joke that the only difference between the workers and the patients is that the patients got better," she said.

"Not all of them did," I told her. "Nancy died two years after she left that place."

"Suicide?" she wanted to know.

"Yes," I said.

Ursula paused. "Hmmm. Ouch."

THE MOST DELIGHTFUL PART of piecing together our family story was tracking down Nancy's and Danny's old friends. I missed them! And they missed me. We were so excited to talk to each other that we kept interrupting one another.

We called each other by our old nicknames and remembered funny stories and familiar landmarks. Danny's friend Mike—a.k.a. Plumb Guy—recalled the greasy spoon where he and Danny would fill up on cheeseburgers after mowing lawns. Nancy's old high school boyfriend, the one Holmer nicknamed "the Kisser," told me about making out with Nancy by the rocks at Gillson Park and how she slapped back his advance when he tried getting to "second base" in the back of his steamy Camaro. *I'm not ready for that yet,* she told him. *But, when I am, you'll be the first to know.* Inside jokes came rolling off our tongues like we'd just seen each other last week.

It shocked me to think of them as they are now. Nancy's pals are grandparents about to turn seventy. Danny's old friends are considering retirement as they approach their sixtieth birthdays. As we talked, we were transported back to our teenage days with all the hopes and possibilities that time offered.

Over the years, vestiges of Nancy and Danny will surface, like sparks through stubble, as ghostly reminders of how lively they once were. I'm scrolling through Facebook and suddenly—boom!—there's Danny, walking across my computer screen, winking at me from beyond the grave. One of his old classmates has posted a video from their St. Francis graduation in 1977, decades before Facebook was invented. I hit Replay over and over, soaking up every second of watching my little brother flash a devilish grin.

My phone dings, and I open a text to find Nancy's face staring at me. My friend Terry found Nancy's old University of Colorado student ID while leafing through an old photo album. Nancy gave it to her when we were in college so Terry could use it as a fake ID to buy beer.

These unexpected images of Nancy and Danny make me gasp. They look so young! Their eyes sparkle. Their thick, dark hair shines. They are frozen in time with no hints of the ravages of our old age—crow's feet, sagging jowls, aching joints, streaks of gray hair. They never had the chance to get old.

When someone dies suddenly, especially if it's by suicide, you don't get to grieve them in the same way that you do for someone who's lived a full life or battled a long illness. You might strain to recall an amusing anecdote or two, but to assuage the guilt or dull the shock, you constantly remind yourself how sick they were and that they are much better off now that they are dead.

That fixed narrative made it easier for us, but it also overshadowed the quirks and qualities that made Nancy and Danny so dynamic. Talking to Danny's and Nancy's friends helped me to remember them in all the endearing ways I would not allow myself to consider I had forgotten how Nancy used to shout, "See food!" and then open her mouth to show you what she was chewing or the way Danny would turn his head suddenly and repeat his favorite *Caddyshack* line: "How about a Fresca?"

Danny's friend Sully told me a hilarious story about the night Danny tied a rope from his motorboat around his waist and lugged the vessel along the shores of Lake Michigan with many of his workers on board. His college buddy Norm recalled how Danny rounded up three of his friends on a lark one night and drove straight through to Providence, Rhode Island, to cheer on their Loyola Rambler basketball team. Hearing about their antics—how Nancy practiced talking to boys in the mirror, Danny's perfect Neil Young impression—brought their spirits back to life so that I had to stop every now and then to remind myself that they are long dead.

You can't find peace without properly grieving, and we—or at least

I—had not allowed ourselves to sit with our sadness, to acknowledge the sorrow of these two beautiful people dying so young.

I found Nancy's old pal Joy where all grandmothers live these days—on Facebook. We met in the restaurant of a hotel near where one of her grandsons was playing hockey. Joy and Nancy were close in high school and stayed friends through their first year of college. She scared the hell out of me back then, with her foul mouth and wilting stare.

Joy and I had not seen one another in fifty years, but I was still nervous to meet with her. Funny how those old dynamics linger. I was curious to know what she remembered about my sister. Between my decision to avoid Nancy in the years leading up to her death and the trauma of her suicide, I could barely recall anything about my sister anymore. I clung to whatever earthly possessions might keep us linked, refusing to throw out her old red ski jacket, for instance. But, with each passing year, a little more of Nancy faded from my mind. I was hoping that Joy might have some memories that would trigger a few of my own.

She was able to recall a few snippets, like how Nancy loaned her a dress for a sock hop and helped her with her makeup. But nothing she said sparked much to help me remember Nancy better.

"Those were our hippie days," Joy said. "Lots of drugs and stuff like that."

Joy went to college in Denver and visited Nancy a few times in Boulder, but they lost touch after Nancy's car crash. Joy can't remember when or how she heard that Nancy died.

"I remember writing a note to your dad when I heard about it," she said.

Regardless of Joy's faint memory, it felt good just to be sitting and talking to someone who knew my sister. After forty years of sobriety, Joy seemed to be a lot kinder and more approachable than the surly teenager I once dreaded. We chatted easily. She was funny and sweet. I didn't want to leave. I kept looking at Joy and wondering how she had managed to get her life together when Nancy could not. Why do some people recover but others don't?

Oddly, I found myself confessing to Joy, saying the things I wish I could have said to Nancy, as though she were her surrogate. I told Joy how guilty I felt about all the lost opportunities to connect with my sister in the final years of her life. I described how I visited Nancy in the psych ward at Evanston Hospital a week after she tried drowning herself in the bathtub and how I got up to leave without saying goodbye because I was angry at how rude I thought she was being to me. I should have understood that Nancy was terribly depressed, I told Joy. I wish I had told her that I was sorry that she was feeling so lost and hopeless.

"Nancy was sick, and I treated her like shit," I told Joy. "I'm afraid I wasn't a very good sister to her."

Joy shook her head and waved her hand for me to stop.

"You couldn't have gotten to her," Joy said. "No one could."

It felt good to vent, to say these things out loud.

Joy cleared her throat. She had something to tell me.

A friend of hers had a party recently where a psychic was giving readings and "it was kinda fun," Joy said. So she made an appointment with her to ask about Nancy, knowing that the two of us would be meeting.

Oh, boy, I thought. *This conversation might be getting a little too weird.* I didn't really believe in the power of the supernatural, but I confess that I was eager to hear what this woman had to say about Nancy.

"She said Nancy was laughing," Joy told me. "She was with your mother and father and they had a dog. Nancy wanted you to know that she is doing good."

A dog?

Joy leaned in and continued in her thick Chicago accent. "She said, 'Don't worry about me. It was nobody's fault. I'm fine.'" I could feel tears pooling in my eyes, and I started to blink. I hadn't cried about my sister in years.

"Nancy has a message specifically for you," Joy said.

"She said, 'Tell my sister that I've been there all along, during her graduation from college, at her wedding, the whole thing.' Whenever you see one of those little glints of light, like on a prism, the kind that shines in your eyes? That's Nancy. She's reaching out to you."

It didn't matter to me if what this psychic was saying was true or not, though I wished that it were. Just the notion that my sister's old friend—the one who used to make me so nervous—was now going to great lengths to comfort me felt liberating. It was as if Nancy was forgiving me through Joy. I started to weep.

"I'm sorry," I told Joy, fumbling in my pocket for a Kleenex.

We had been talking for more than an hour. I could have stayed there all day, hungry as I was for any connection to Nancy, but Joy needed to get to her grandson's game.

"Wait. I've got something for you," she said, digging into her purse. Joy pulled out a little plastic angel the size of a pecan. It was wrapped in cellophane. She handed it to me as we stood to leave. As I unwrapped it, I could see that the little angel's wings were sprinkled with glitter that sparkled like tiny prisms of light.

MY BIGGEST COUP WAS finding our old live-in babysitter from 1960 to 1962. I was three and four years old when she lived with us, and now all I could remember was her maiden name, the last name of her first husband, and that she reminded me of Connie Francis from *Where the Boys Are*.

In exchange for room and board, Linda, a student at a college nearby, helped my mother each weeknight feed us dinner and get us off to bed. The alumni office at the former National College of Education, now known as National Louis University, was closed during the early days of the pandemic. But several months later, they emailed me to say that they had tracked down her address in Florida. I called and left a message on what I hoped was her answering machine. "Don't faint," I said, giving my name and the reason for my call. "I'm hoping you can help me fill in some blanks." Linda called me back two days later while I was strolling my baby granddaughter around a park in Connecticut. Would she even remember us? Even after sixty years, Linda didn't skip a beat.

"If I had a pencil and paper, I could draw all of your faces this minute," she said. "The two years I spent with your family were two of the happiest years of my life." Her words floored me. I'd always considered my family to be joyful and fun to be around, despite our tragedies. Now, here was validation.

She recalled Patty's curly hair and what a "little gentleman" Jake was. Nancy was quiet and studious and "smart as a whip" and Mary Kay was cute and helpful. She wanted to know if Billy was "still such a rascal."

A farm girl from Michigan, Linda had been studying to become a teacher, and she practiced her techniques on us. She brought our art projects for the rest of the class to analyze.

"There were so many of you, I could do all my research right there in your playroom," she said. Linda and my mother did their best to pick up the house each afternoon that Holmer was in town before he walked in the door from work.

"Your dad could be tough," she said. "He wanted those floors to be clean."

My mother was kind and funny and easy to be with, Linda said. There was one quality of my mother's that struck Linda as odd.

"She loved getting her hair done more than anyone I've ever known."

She was sad and surprised to learn what happened to Nancy and Danny. She never thought of our family as troubled or strange.

"The one word I would use to describe you all was *normal*," Linda said. "You were all such good, happy kids, and good to one another."

But she was not surprised to hear about my mother's breakdown after we moved back from New Canaan.

"She didn't want to go," Linda said. "Can you imagine how hard that must have been for her?"

I wondered if they ever discussed my mother's depression and anxiety. "People didn't talk about those things then," she said. But Linda could see that my mother struggled and that we wore her out. "Even though she loved each of you and really enjoyed being with you, she'd get so tired."

Families are complicated. Then she told me a bit about what had gone on in hers. She wished me luck and assured me that, whatever else I found out, this was the most important thing to know:

"There was a lot of love in that house," Linda said. "A lot of love."

18

Pillars of Light

We are all brothers, and we are all suffering from the same fate. The same smoke floats over all our heads. Help one another. It is the only way to survive.

—ELIE WIESEL, *Night*

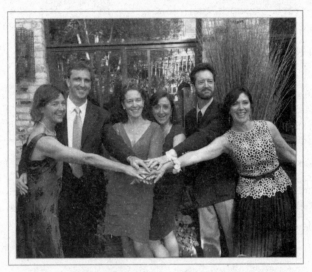

All for one, and one for all. Chicago, 2014: Molly, Billy, Patty, me, Jake, and Mary Kay.

Our Kissinger family text chain has gotten out of control. It began innocently enough with the usual happy birthday, happy anniversary, merry Christmas messages. Next came the occasional politically motivated rants, which seem to have mellowed since the 2020 presidential election. And, of course, news flashes. When a relative or someone from the old neighborhood dies, we send out an APB under the headline: "Guess Who Can't Come to the Phone Anymore?" Increasingly, we are sending goofy memes, heavy on themes involving *Seinfeld,* *Caddyshack,* and *The Office.* Now my nephew Ryan has taken to texting us each time he comes across a name suggestive of a phallus, like Harry Sackrider or former Chicago Cub Pete LaCock.

We can't stop trying to make each other laugh. It's gotten to the point where those of us with day jobs have to silence our notifications.

On family Zoom calls, we talk over each other so much, it's hard to follow the conversations. The in-laws and our kids and grandkids have learned to make quick cameos and leave the jibber-jabber to us siblings, the Original Gangsters, or OGs, as we now call ourselves.

Likewise, when one of us lands in the hospital, whether it's for colon cancer or a new hip or bronchitis, we drop everything and rally. For a family once scattered and torn apart by mental illness, we've grown quite tribal, very protective. We're back piling on top of each other in a virtual game of Teddy Bear, our old playroom family classic.

When matters are graver—one of our kids won't get out of bed or is drinking too much—we'll pick up the phone and call each other for advice or consolation or just to vent. We are very protective of this next generation and, knowing our family history, we have good reason to be. We aren't silent any longer, sharing tips and resources.

Bipolar disorder and depression run in families. They certainly do in ours. The kids of our next generation have struggled, too, some with anxiety, others with depression and bipolar disorder. Some have had issues with substance abuse, eating disorders, even our greatest fear: thoughts of suicide. Is it nature or nurture? The role that genes play is still not fully understood. But we now know that trauma passed down from one generation to the next and environmental factors like stress and drug and alcohol abuse can trigger symptoms.

We dream about the day some scientist will figure out a blood test or some kind of scan that identifies people with mental illness so they can get help before their illnesses get out of control. We fantasize about what it would be like to swallow a pill and be cured.

That day will never come without a greater commitment by the scientific community and government funders. Just 4 percent of the world's health research funding was spent on mental illnesses from 2015 to 2019, a study in *The Lancet Psychiatry* found. Even the normally reserved authors called that "pathetic." Spending on research for a cause and cure for bipolar, aka the Kissinger curse, is even worse. A 2021 review by the Treatment Advocacy Center found that federal funding for bipolar research lags well behind other serious mental illnesses. Several years ago, we got excited about the research into the MTHFR gene mutation (which we called the "Motherfucker gene") associated with depression and anxiety. A few of us have been tested and found to have the mutation. But this is far from an explanation of how or even if the gene causes mental illness. It certainly does not offer a cure.

Despite this, we have lots of reasons to be hopeful. People living with mental illness have so many more resources now than we did when we were growing up: Social/emotional learning, robust mental health advocacy organizations, a dedicated national suicide prevention hotline. I am heartened to see how my students' and my kids' generations are so much more willing to discuss their mental health and ask for help. They counsel and console each other in ways that we never did.

Research shows that integrating family with treatment is leading to fewer psychotic episodes, fewer hospital admissions, and better engagement with treatment. When family gets involved in the treatment, the patient is more likely to have a better mood, a richer quality of life, enhanced work performance, and reduced substance use.

If Nancy were a teenager today, she would have a much better chance at surviving. Her medications would be better. She would have access to more robust therapy. Likely, we would have gotten family therapy. We would be more willing and better able to talk to her about her feelings and ours. If nothing else, she might have found a group of kindred spirits on social media.

Ditto for Danny. Some high school counselor probably would have been assigned to help him after Nancy died. He would have healthier

ways to process her death. We all would have. We would be better versed
in knowing the signs of bipolar disorder and what to do when someone
becomes obsessive and paranoid.

Of course, I can't say that Nancy and Danny would not still have taken
their own lives, but we surely would have been more proactive about
helping them.

Still, much more work needs to be done. The suicide rate in the United
States is up more than 35 percent since 1997, the year that Danny died.
That's not a typo. Thirty-five percent. This comes as the rate in other
Western nations has fallen. Experts say this most likely is because we have
become a more isolated society, paradoxically even as social media makes
us better able to connect with one another.

Prevention experts have identified several factors that add to the risk of
suicide: violence in the home, financial insecurity, access to lethal means,
lack of coping skills, isolation, previous attempts. We had all of these.

Suicide is preventable, the experts say. It starts by talking about it.

THE FIRST HALF OF Mary Oliver's poem that guided me as I wrote this
book reads:

> *Look, the trees*
> *are turning*
> *their own bodies*
> *into pillars*
>
> *of light,*
> *are giving off the rich*
> *fragrance of cinnamon*
> *and fulfillment*

That is what has happened to us. We have become our own pillars of
light.

Mary Kay found her art, Jake, his support groups, I had my journalism,

Patty, her science. Billy turned to music and Molly to the mountains and the sea. We each found a place where we could try to make sense of the trauma of our past and find a way to reconcile it.

I knew when I started to write this book that there was a lot I could learn about those who died. But I also knew that I had just as much to learn from the ones who lived. I watched over the years as my brothers and sisters each found their footing and went on to build rich, rewarding lives.

Mary Kay is an artist in Chicago. Jake works as an inventory manager at an electrical supply company. Patty is an epidemiologist and associate dean at Tulane University's School of Public Health & Tropical Medicine. Billy writes news stories for WGN-TV in Chicago. Molly coaches volleyball and teaches yoga and kiteboarding in Mexico and Oregon.

I asked each of them what advice they would offer families that have lost someone to suicide. They all stressed the need for counseling.

"Try for family therapy, but if you get resistance, get help for yourself," Mary Kay said. She suggested the American Foundation for Suicide Prevention and the National Alliance on Mental Illness.

Jake warned that it might take a while for therapy or self-help groups to work.

"Go even if they don't make you feel better at first," Jake said. "Give them a chance to work." Ever the practical thinker, Jake added this shiny pearl of wisdom: "Have a good picture of the person who died."

Patty, who spent a decade in Africa and Haiti, said she learned firsthand that avoidance "only works for so long." Ultimately, she turned to therapy to help understand her feelings about what went on in our house "and I am still working through it." She reminded people who have been through the suicide of someone they love to remember that it is not your fault. "Keep taking care of yourself and speak frankly about it."

Anyone affected by suicide needs a lot of support. "The less stigma there is in talking about it, the healthier we will be," Patty said.

Everyone agreed that living with someone in the throes of severe mental illness is difficult. Billy advised being as patient and understanding as possible but warned, "Mental illness can be mean and ugly." Walk away when it gets too rough, if you can. "Don't allow the person to abuse you," he said. "You just have to play zone defense and contain it" as best as you are able. Having a sense of humor is helpful, too, Billy said. "Not to be flippant or dismissive but just as a reminder that our time is limited and precious and shouldn't be lived wallowing in misery and self-pity."

Find a way to carve out some place where you can be at peace, Molly said. She has relied heavily on nature and physical activity—swimming, basketball, tennis, volleyball, skiing, wind sports, and yoga. She also read lots of self-help books and sought counseling whenever she could. "Practice daily self-care," she said. "One breath at a time. Resilience is a full-spectrum, long, slow, curious process."

Be mindful, Molly said. "Find something to be grateful for each day when you wake up. Practice forgiveness."

As I was finishing writing this book, I got an email from a woman I had written about twelve years earlier. Truthfully, I barely remembered her. She had filed a complaint against her Wisconsin psychiatrist in 2010, claiming he had sexually abused her years earlier. The psychiatrist was being accused of mishandling other cases at the Milwaukee County Mental Health Complex.

Her email to me in the spring of 2022 came out of the blue, as I had not heard from her since my story about her ran. I was so busy chronicling one shocking example of mistreatment and abuse after another back then that the stories started to blend together. When I think about those days now, I'm sure I was suffering from some post-traumatic stress of my own. So, getting this email from her more than a decade later was a jolt.

"I've read most of your articles and remember that you lost a loved one to suicide," she wrote. She added a link to the American Foundation for Suicide Prevention and a fundraising walk they were sponsoring.

"I'm walking to honor your brother," she wrote.

I was so touched by her thoughtfulness that I asked if I could call her. When we spoke the next day, I learned that she was a doctor working in New York City, not far from where I teach. I told her that my students are always curious about the best ways to interview what we call "sensitive subjects," those like her who have been victims of sexual abuse or other forms of trauma. Would she be able to help me brainstorm what to tell them based on her experience of coming forward with her story?

They're so worried about not wanting to hurt the person they are interviewing, I said, recalling my own trepidation when I interviewed her more than a decade earlier.

Tell them it is going to hurt, she said. *That's how the healing starts.*

She began her career as a doctor treating AIDS patients in the Bronx at the height of that epidemic. Nearly every day, she had to be the one to break the news to patients who had been diagnosed with what was then almost certainly a death sentence. The average life span of a person diagnosed with AIDS in the late 1980s was eighteen months. This woman, now in her midsixties, supervises medical residents in New York.

She trains her students to ask clear, probing questions to make a proper diagnosis. Often, she says, that means the patient will experience some embarrassment, even pain.

I loved that advice and was delighted when she agreed to come to my class.

My students were as impressed as I had been at her courage to come forward, both in meeting with us and, years earlier, when she filed her complaint against her psychiatrist. She knew she would be risking backlash, possible exposure and pushback from the psychiatrist who had abused her, reopening those old wounds.

What motivated you to take this risk? One of my students asked. The woman paused for a bit and then told them about an exhibit she had seen many years ago at New York's Museum of Arts and Design. Green Guerillas, the environmental advocacy group, had taken a limb from a tree that had been killed by pesticides and decorated it in glitter.

This is what telling your story can do, she told them. It can bring the dead back to life—not in the same way but as a kind of transformation. It doesn't take away the injury, but it can give you a feeling of power when you are in control of the narrative. The balance is shifted back to you. There's new life, resurrected.

That is what writing this book has done for me. It gave me a framework for confronting my demons, staring down my past to make peace with it. For so many years, I had identified myself by my family's tragedies, stuck in the mindset of the daughter of two lovable but deeply troubled souls, the sister who lost two siblings to suicide. More than wife or mother or, now, grandmother. More than a reporter or professor or friend. I was defining myself by events in my life that I had no control over.

I watched in gratitude as my siblings came forward, one by one, to share their stories of resilience and recovery, trusting me to tell our family's story in the most public way. Each of us has tanked at one time or another. We have all been dangerously close to losing control, feeling waves of sadness that we could not explain or will away. But we each found ways to cope. Eventually, we—even I, the one who has spent a whole career writing about other people's mental illness—found power in asking questions and telling our stories. No more *if anyone asks, this was an accident*. Now, if anyone asks, this is what really happened.

Slowly, the choke hold of those traumas has begun to loosen. That's not to say that we don't struggle from time to time. But we are no longer ashamed to admit that.

The ones in the next generation are doing what they can to make a diagnosis of mental illness better understood and less shameful. My daughter, Molly, got her graduate degree in risk prevention from Harvard University's Graduate School of Education and for more than a decade has been working in student mental health outreach and support. Billy's daughter, Cayleigh, is studying psychology with hopes of becoming a counselor. All our children are passionate advocates for better mental health.

I USED TO THINK we could conquer mental illness by beating it into submission, the way Patty and I imagined pounding the tigers that we thought swirled beneath our twin beds. Now I see that we need to make peace with the fact that mental illness is a lifetime struggle. It will always be with us. We have to find ways to live with it, embrace it and one another. Acknowledge that we are human, that we all suffer. When we accept that, we demystify mental illness and strip it of its power to tear us apart.

Jake is living proof that someone with a serious mental illness can live a good life. He suffers but is well loved and is loving in return. He is a valued employee, a treasured friend and housemate, and now, our cherished patriarch.

Jake reaches out to us when he is feeling depressed or having especially disturbing thoughts, and we jump. He recently sent us all a text saying he was having a hard time packing for our family reunion in Saugatuck, Michigan. Would someone please call him to help? By the time I saw the message five minutes later and called him, he had just gotten off the phone with Patty. After Jake and I hung up, Molly called.

With lots of work and the help of those around us, we are learning how to live alongside the tigers, to put ourselves back together again. We are telling our story and letting go.

A FEW YEARS AFTER Danny died, I asked Holmer if he ever regretted *not* playing the Get Out of Jail Free card that my mother had offered him just weeks before their wedding. We were sitting next to each other on an airplane, on our way to Ireland to meet Patty and Molly for some laughs, a trip that none of us could really afford but all of us felt we dearly needed. The gut punch of losing Danny had left us reeling. Ten days hiking in that grand old land of our ancestors, with its rocky coasts and quaint pubs, would do wonders for our spirits, as it had for Mary Kay, Patty, and me twenty years earlier, not long after Nancy died.

I thought about the story of how my parents' wedding was nearly canceled and wondered how close we came to never having been born at all.

My mother figured that, with her anxiety and Holmer's wild mood swings, the two of them probably should not get married and start a family. She knew that raising children would be a lot of responsibility, and she worried that the two of them might not be able to handle it well. Her hesitation seemed more like a premonition to me now.

Was it worth it? I asked Holmer.

It was a fair question, considering how everything had turned out. Knowing then what he knows now, would he still have gone ahead and married my mother? Should he have? Should this family have come into being in the first place?

The minute I blurted it out, I feared the answer.

Part of me was hoping that Holmer would jump at the answer to my existential question. *Of course I'm glad I married your mother, stupid!* I thought he might say. *Sure, we've had terrible sorrow, but look at all the laughs we've had—and still have. I wouldn't trade those good times for anything. Love is our greatest treasure. The sting of its loss is the price we must pay.*

But another part of me worried that he might say no, that he would have been better off taking his chances with someone else. The pain of watching his children suffer and die had been too much for him to bear. And for the rest of us, for that matter.

Holmer closed his eyes for a minute and smiled wistfully. Then he leaned his head against the window and turned his face toward the black night as the sea roared thousands of feet below us. If he said something, I didn't hear it. I considered repeating my question but decided against it.

Did I really want to know if my father regretted marrying my mother or if he was sorry that my siblings and I had ever been born? It wasn't going to change what happened. For once in my life, I was relieved not to have the answer, if there was one at all.

Some things are best left a mystery.

Look, the trees
are turning
their own bodies
into pillars

of light,
are giving off the rich
fragrance of cinnamon
and fulfillment,

the long taper
of cattails
are bursting and floating away over
the blue shoulders

of the ponds,
and every pond,
no matter what its
name is, is

nameless now.
Every year
everything
I have ever learned

in my lifetime
leads back to this: the fires
and the black river of loss
whose other side

is salvation,
whose meaning
none of us will ever know.
To live in this world

you must be able
to do three things:

to love what is mortal;
to hold it

against your bones knowing
your own life depends on it;
and, when the time comes to let it
go,
to let it go.
—MARY OLIVER, *In Blackwater Woods*

Acknowledgments

The problem with thanking people who have helped me with this book is that it's like eating a bite of mint chocolate-chip ice cream: once I start, I don't want to stop. So, let me begin with an apology to anyone I've forgotten to mention here, because I know you are out there.

So many people helped me with this book, but no one more than Larry Boynton, my life raft / husband / personal chef / typo catcher / wilderness guide. Too bad you don't believe in saints, because you are one. Our loving and brilliant children, Charley and Molly—promise me that you'll wait until I'm dead to write your memoirs. God knows I've given you enough material. Sawyer Emmer, my hilarious son-in-law, and his little sunshine crew, Winnie and Dot. Gram Gram loves you.

This book could not have been written without the help of my brave, generous, clever brothers and sisters: Mary Kay, Jake, Patty, Billy, and Molly. The best part about writing this book was getting to spend time with you, remembering Nancy and Danny and Holmer and our mom. I'm grateful to the spouses and partners, Tom Warden, Annie Kerwin, Michael Perlstein, Dana Kozlov, and Kenny Bresnihan and my sassy/adorable nieces and nephews, Ryan, Connor, Devin, Max, Eli, Jackie, Cayleigh, Brennan, Leo, Mary Rose, and Patrick. This is your story, too. SUCH a funny family.

Shout-out to our cousins the Dorwards; the McIntyres, especially Mike

McIntyre for his tireless cheerleading; the Gutenkunsts, especially Dodie and Heidi; and Mary Jo Gerlach, who helped me research family stories. Special props to Jim Ritter, whose early read and keen questions helped shape this book. I also want to thank my Boynton family cheering section—my talented sisters-in-law Betsy Killorin and Cia Ochsenbein; Cia's husband, Roland; and Betsy's kids, Andy, Abby, and Sam.

I'm most grateful to my skillful editors, Jamie Raab and Cecily van Buren-Freedman. They saw that this could be a book someday and deftly coaxed it out of me. Gail Ross, my agent, and her talented assistant, Dara Kaye, shined up my proposal well enough to catch Jamie's eye. Kate Greenway, my thoughtful and insightful therapist, steadied me and helped me tiptoe through the minefield of my life so that I could make good on my pledge: No Kissingers were harmed in the making of this book!

Eternal gratitude and admiration to the families who shared their frustrations and sorrows with me over the years and modeled what true love looks like under the most challenging conditions, especially the Spoerl family—Pat, Joe Jr., Margie, and Joan—Georgia Rawlings's family—Jeanne, Debbie, and Ted—Debbie Sweeney, Rob Sweeney, Amanda Farrell, Helen Kriewaldt, Mike and Kathy Weigl, Myron and Jean Anczak, and Kathy Despears.

My deepest thanks to those from way back who helped me resurrect the spirits of Nancy and Danny: Linda Engel, Joe Eberle, Mike Plumb, Ted Perry, Norm Labrasca, Patrick Sullivan, Tom Dieschbourg, Jack Storer, Shotsi Cain Lajoie, Chris Kysar, Joy Bowler Sheldon, and Ellen Cordell.

So much of the material for this book came from stories that I reported for the *Milwaukee Journal Sentinel*. I was fortunate to work with some of the best editors and reporters in the world there: George Stanley, Marty Kaiser, Greg Borowski, Mike Juley, Becky Lang, Tom Koetting, and David Haynes. Margo Huston showed me how to write about people with dignity and compassion and told me about that beautiful Mary Oliver poem. Thanks too to Steve Schultze and Dave Umhoefer, who insisted that I write this book. My outrageously entertaining crew from the *Journal Sentinel* lunch table kept me laughing: Susanne Rust, Rick Romell,

Jim Stingl, Dan Egan, Crocker Stephenson, and John Fauber. Thanks, too, to photographers and graphic designers Gary Porter, Lou Saldivar, and Kris Wentz, for their wizardry.

Celestial shout-out to those dear newsroom friends who inspired me but are now gone: Tim Cuprisin, Don Walker, Whitney Gould, and Meg Jones.

Thanks to my old Watertown pals Bob Diddlebock and John B. Johnson. Shout-out to my old *Cincinnati Post* editor Mike O'Connor, who got me to believe in myself. Thanks to my Milwaukee writing group: Martha Bergland, Barbara Miner, Terri Sutton, and Doug Armstrong. Thanks also to my Milwaukee book group, aka The Fanny Flag Fan Club: Mary Ann Klabunde, Lucy Berman-Edelman, Sharon Moore, Amy Daniels, Andrea Wagoner, Marie Beduhn, Ginny Stoffel, and the late Connie Mullins.

Love to my Pomodoro pal and former student, Gina Ryder, who helped me from start to finish, and to Laura Muha, who cheered me, especially in those early days. Thanks to Lili Wright, who let me sit in on her senior seminar at DePauw University, and the legendary Samuel Freedman, who allowed me to audit his famous book proposal class at Columbia Journalism School.

I'm grateful to all I learned from the dozens of brilliant students I taught over the years at Columbia University and to the fearless and talented journalists and mental health professionals who helped us understand the system and its failings: Bob Kolker, Jason Cherkis, Megan Twohey, Gabriel Dance, Ellen Gabler, Pam Belluck, Rob Waters, John Ackerman, Alana Mendelsohn, Linda Rosenberg, Deborah Doroshow, Lloyd Sederer, Charles Ornstein, Glenn Speer, Christopher Magoon, Rachel Aviv, Anne Harrington, Taylor Eldridge, Stephen Fried, Sean Campbell, Ben Carey, Caitlin McCarthy, Mary Cregan, Zack McDermott, Michael Ray, Oriana Zill de Granados, Ali Mattu, Lise Zumwalt, Alisa Roth, Kenneth Paul Rosenberg, Mustafa Mirza, Sarah Smith, John Snook, Jeannie Vanasco, Heather Schroering, Adiel Kaplan, the good people at the Rosalynn Carter Center for Mental Health Journalism, the Treatment Advocacy Center, the Bazelon Center for Mental Health Law, the Solutions Journalism Network, and Columbia's Dart Center.

Fact: This book would not have happened without the encouragement of Tom Jennings, a genius and real cool cat, who helped me find an agent and smoothed the way for me to a Logan writing fellowship. All hail Carly Willsie and the whole gang at the Logan Nonfiction Program, a modern-day Eden, and the talented band of inspiring wordsmiths I met there, particularly Stobo Sniderman, Susan Berfield, Amy Marcus, and Pat Evangelista.

Special thanks to my trusty researcher Khaya Himmelman, who found some eye-popping facts, and early readers Elizabeth Janowski, Justin Lynch, David Jeans, Temima Shulman, Casey Parks, Amanda Darrach, Olivia Carville, Isabel Ruehl, and Ian Halim.

Thanks to Marion Roach Smith, whose Memoir Project became a kind of bible. To Mike Byrne and Jim Crowley, esquires at law and all-around good guys, who helped me get my family's medical records.

To my lifelong pals Mary Claire Compernolle Belton, Terry Byrne Broccolo, Beth Pritchard Kerr, Patti Maloney, and Jane Brazes Funke, who have always been there for me. Love you ladies so much.

Woot woot to the Alice Egan family, particularly Alice and Sarah, who read early versions. My walking buddies and neighbors kept me chugging—Marcy Keefe, Laurie Segal, Katie Roozen, Ellie Tucker, Deb Goldin, Joan Balliet, and Kathy Albright—and my Lake Michigan plunging pals Shelly Weingarten, Vicki O'Neill, Kate Christensen, and Christy Moser, aka the Hardy Girls.

If this were the Academy Awards, they would have played me off the stage by now. Just know that I am one lucky dog to have had so many wonderful people who've helped me get this book out of my body and into the world. Finally, thanks to Sister Mary Assisi, who knew I was hurting and treated me kindly; Eve Sylvester, who prayed for me; all the angels and saints in heaven and, of course, my guardian angel. I promise to always make room for you wherever I go.

Notes

Front Matter General

xii   **There's also the matter of trauma:** Kristin W. Samuelson, "Post-Traumatic Stress Disorder and Declarative Memory Functioning: A Review." *Dialogues in Clinical Neuroscience* 13, no. 3 (2011): 346–51, https://www.ncbi.nlm.nih.gov/pmc/articles/PMC3182004/.

1. The Tiger Pit

4   **"Something is definitely wrong":** Judith Blake, "The Americanization of Catholic Reproductive Ideals," *Population Studies* 20, no. 1 (1966): 27–43, doi: 10.1080/00324728.1966.10406082.

2. Get Out of Jail Free

25   **Decades later, it would be revealed:** Robert Blanchard, "Sobering Stats: 15,000 U.S. Airmen Killed in Training in WW II," Real Clear History, Feb. 12, 2019, https://www.realclearhistory.com/articles/2019/02/12/staggering_statistics_15000_us_airmen_killed_in_training_in_ww_ii_412.html; Marlyn R. Pierce, "Earning Their Wings: Accidents and Fatalities in the United States Army Air Forces During Flight Training in World War Two," doctoral dissertation, Kansas State University, Manhattan, KS, 2013, https://core.ac.uk/download/pdf/18529342.pdf.

27   **Nearly half died in the first year:** A. H. Bittles and E. J. Glasson, "Clinical, Social, and Ethical Implications of Changing Life Expectancy in Down Syndrome," *Developmental Medicine & Child Neurology* 46 (2004): 282–86, https://onlinelibrary.wiley.com/doi/pdf/10.1111/j.1469-8749.2004.tb00483.x.

32   **More than 35 million prescriptions:** Andrea Tone, "Listening to the Past: History, Psychiatry, and Anxiety," *Canadian Journal of Psychiatry* 50, no. 7 (June 2005): 373–80, https://journals.sagepub.com/doi/pdf/10.1177/070674370505000702.

5. It's All in Her Head

65   **A fungal infection:** "Dutch Elm Disease," Village of Wilmette, https://www.wilmette.com /engineering-public-works/forestry/dutch-elm-disease/.

9. Love and a Hate Crime

142   **The group chose that venue:** Chris Demaske, "Village of Skokie v. National Socialist Party of America (Ill) (1978)," The First Amendment Encyclopedia (2009), https://www.mtsu.edu/first -amendment/article/728/village-of-skokie-v-national-socialist-party-of-america-ill.

12. Collecting Treasures for Heaven

190   **Biblical scholars consider Job:** Mike Bennett, "The Book of Job," Life, Hope & Truth, https:// lifehopeandtruth.com/bible/holy-bible/old-testament/the-writings/job/.

13. Swimming Back to Devil's Island

199   **My focus was on the much smaller subset:** National Institute of Mental Health, "Mental Illness," https://www.nimh.nih.gov/health/statistics/mental-illness#part_154788.

200   **More than one-third:** Substance Abuse and Mental Health Services Administration, "Key Substance Use and Mental Health Indicators in the United States: Results from the 2019 National Survey on Drug Use and Health" (2020), https://www.samhsa.gov/data/sites/default/files /reports/rpt29393/2019NSDUHFFRPDFWHTML/2019NSDUHFFR1PDFW090120.pdf.

200   **A person with serious mental illness:** Prison Policy Initiative, "Mental Health," https://www .prisonpolicy.org/research/mental_health/.

200   **More than a quarter:** National Coalition for the Homeless, "Mental Illness and Homelessness," July 2009, https://www.nationalhomeless.org/factsheets/Mental_Illness.pdf.

200   **Their average life span:** Megan Hull, "Poor Mental Health's Devastating Impacts on Life Expectancy—And How Treatment Can Help," Recovery Village, updated April 28, 2022, https:// www.therecoveryvillage.com/mental-health/mental-health-impact-on-life-expectancy/#:~:text =According%20to%20the%20World%20Health,year%20reduction%20in%20life%20expectancy.

203   **The orderlies were shocked:** NPR, "WWII Pacifists Exposed Mental Ward Horrors," *All Things Considered*, Dec. 30, 2009, https://www.npr.org/2009/12/30/122017757/wwii -pacifists-exposed-mental-ward-horrors.

204   **In the end, fewer than half:** Shannon Bradford, "The History of Community Mental Health Care," *Chicago Policy Review*, March 12, 2021, https://chicagopolicyreview.org/2021/03/12 /community-mental-health-care-lessons-from-history.

15. Holmer in the Gloamin'

233   **The cause for her optimism:** Meg Kissinger, "Meg Kissinger Thursday Chat Transcript," *Milwaukee Journal Sentinel*, Dec. 15, 2011, https://archive.jsonline.com/news/health/135305763 .html/.

17. Like Sparks Through Stubble

272 **I had been haunted by a study:** Hull, "Poor Mental Health's Devastating Impacts on Life Expectancy—And How Treatment Can Help."

18. Pillars of Light

286 **Several years ago, we got excited:** Lin Wan, Yuhong Li, Zhengrong Zhang, Zuoli Sun, Yi He, and Rena Li, "Methylenetetrahydrofolate Reductase and Psychiatric Diseases," *Translational Psychiatry* 8 (2018): 242, https://www.ncbi.nlm.nih.gov/pmc/articles/PMC6218441/.

286 **Research shows that integrating family:** Camice J. Revier et al., "Ten-Year Outcomes of First-Episode Psychoses in the MRC ÆSOP-10 Study," *Journal of Nervous and Mental Disease* 203, no. 5 (2015): 379–86, https://www.ncbi.nlm.nih.gov/pmc/articles/PMC4414339/.

287 **The suicide rate in the United States:** National Institute of Mental Health, "Suicide," https://www.nimh.nih.gov/health/statistics/suicide.

About the Author

Meg Kissinger spent more than two decades traveling across the country to report on America's mental health system for the *Milwaukee Journal Sentinel.* A Pulitzer Prize finalist, she has won dozens of accolades, including two George Polk Awards, the Robert F. Kennedy Award, awards from Investigative Reporters and Editors, and two National Journalism Awards. Kissinger teaches investigative reporting at Columbia Journalism School and was a visiting professor at DePauw University, her alma mater. Her stories on the abysmal living conditions for people with mental illness inspired changes to Wisconsin law and led to the creation of hundreds of new housing units. She lives in Milwaukee with her husband.